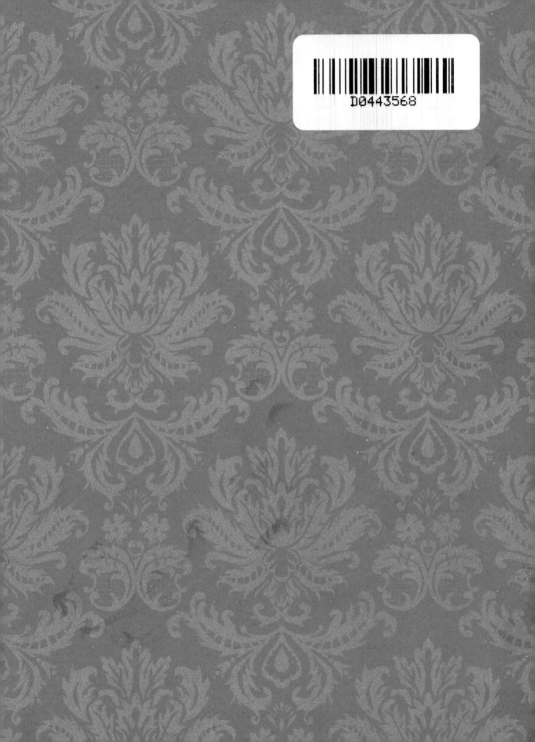

GROWN-UP GLAMOUR

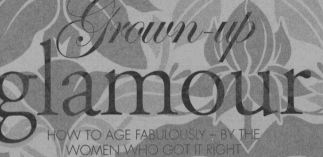

Grown-up glamour

HOW TO AGE FABULOUSLY – BY THE
WOMEN WHO GOT IT RIGHT

CAROLINE COX

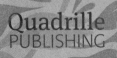

Quadrille
PUBLISHING

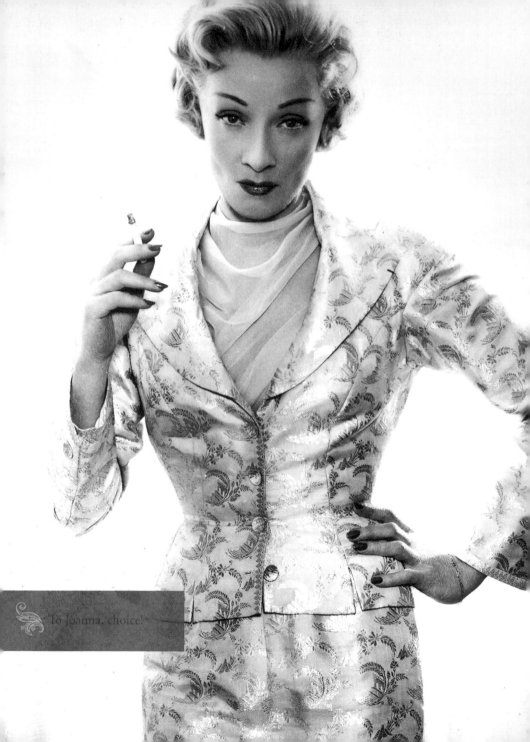

To Joanna, choice!

Marlene Dietrich always demanded a full length mirror next to the camera. With a light directly over her head to white out any signs of aging she would strike her pose.

Grown-up Glamour is the ultimate guide for the grown-up girl who wants to live a life of undisputed elegance and sexy savoir-faire. So many of us dread our journey through adulthood, the embarkation on a stark voyage which seems only to call at the dreary ports of Calorific Deprivation, Neurotic Power-Plating and Pensive Meditation – with occasional forays into Botox. Yet there is another way to successfully segue from the fumbling frustrations and fashion faux pas of kidulthood into an enlightened life of easy pleasure, erotic indulgence and singular je ne sais quoi. Within these pithy pages you will find a cornucopia of tips, hints, beauty and fashion advice with which to sustain your innate sense of style, including modern fashion maxims for the gorgeous new you, a comprehensive guide to dressing divinely. You will be exhorted to 'Hold the Botox!' because a series of miraculous make-up tricks will make you look fresher in minutes, without the need for anaesthetic, and key rules will change the way you think about your hair … forever. Once buffed up to a sexy sheen you will learn how to turn all heads, flirt with skill and present yourself in the best possible light in both boardroom … and bedroom.

SUSTAINING YOUR SPOTLIGHT
Camera, lights, action! As a Seventies glamourpuss would say, 'Today is the first day of the rest of your life,' so why not live it with a little languid sophistication? Don't look over your shoulder at the vagaries of adolescence – pull back your shoulders, adjust your Ray-Bans, sashay your way forward and seize the day with your soft and scented hands! Now, we all know it's all too easy to knock back a cocktail of gin and lithium, loll on the sofa and let the worries of the world wash over us. Blurring the edges after a hard day in the city whilst watching the sordid shenanigans of celebrity pond life on the Samsung goggle box is OK once in a while – but too often it can become a tad habit-forming.

Getting back on the radar can lead to all sorts of deliciousness – we have primal forces so let's use them! And take heed if you think you're already complete, that's a fast track to mummification.

THE MYTH OF INVISIBILITY

Every generation of grown-up girls has a myth to contend with. Today's new myth of 'invisibility' suggests that the older a woman becomes, the more disposable she gets – her attractiveness is proportionate to her fertility. As women fade into the background, their reproductive years trailing behind them, men remain sharply in focus – they stay fertile and automatically sexier too. But hold on a minute, that makes Anna Wintour less compelling than Arsene Wenger, Ben Elton more magnetic than Nastassja Kinski, and Sigourney Weaver's fanciability factor nothing compared to the animal pull of Robin Gibb. *Riiight…*

Women are only invisible if they choose to be – and let's face it, some days you want to be and that's fine. But there are many of us who refuse to be defined by such garbage. If you choose to believe in your invisibility because you are delicately ripening, then desist, because you have allowed a myth to change your perception of yourself – a myth that, although insidious, has no basis in fact.

A compelling, sophisticated and alluring woman will remain so whatever her age – think Cate Blanchett, Helen Mirren, Julie Christie, Marlene Dietrich, Audrey Hepburn and Jackie O. These spectacular women provide blueprints for today's grown-up girls that can be followed with confident ease. So if you fear you may be losing your touch when confronted with yet another celebrity style mag filled with Lindsay Lohan's trout pout and Lady Gaga's knickers, don't take solace in inertia – as Katharine Hepburn said, *'If you don't paddle your own canoe you don't move.'*

FIND YOUR STYLE
The New Fashion Maxims

1

Today's frenetic world of fashion is in the midst of a seismic shift: as we get older, we are looking and feeling better than ever and consequently we are keen to sport clothes with sass and sophistication to match our state of mind. We do not want to wear bin-end bargains, elasticated-waist trousers, 'cheerful' prints or, perish the thought, the same clothes as a 17-year-old. Glamorous grown-ups such as Cate Blanchett, Jerry Hall, Helen Mirren and Jennifer Aniston are showing us the way. All these amazing women have the sense to stand back, take a deep breath and look at the bigger picture, sidelining short-term trends in favour of authenticity. Now it's time for the glamorous grown-up within the rest of us to emerge.

It's certainly not a downhill slide when we get older – in fact, it's the reverse. By now, most of us are beginning to know who we are (and if we don't, there's always therapy!). Additionally, we have more confidence, more money, more power and more taste, so it's time to up our game in the fashion stakes rather than bemoan the fact that crop tops are out. To avoid looking – in that dreadful phrase – like 'mutton dressed as lamb', there are some fairly fundamental pointers:

1 Lovely as they are, ignore Chanel's temporary tattoos. Even if they're flying off the shelves and there's a waiting list, that doesn't mean they're for you.

2 If Louis Vuitton thigh-length boots don't look good on Madonna (and she has the legs of an Olympic sprinter), they will not work for you.

3 When even Scarlett Johansson doesn't suit a nose-ring, it's time to remove the one you had done in the festival field of the Second Summer of Love.

4 If Melanie Griffith cares to go out in a low-cut, black lace body-con minidress, shiny black tights and black court shoes, don't think you can do the same! You'll just look cheap and neurotic.

INDIVIDUAL *Glamour*

Take a deep yogic breath, then release… and wave bye-bye to fast fashion throwaways. It's time to re-discover fashion classics, garments instantly recognizable by the attention to fit, cut and detail, as well as the use of beautiful fabrics. Think Catherine Deneuve in a Burberry trench, a pearl-buttoned cardigan in petrol blue and crisply starched pure white shirt, then mix it up with a vintage crocodile clutch or Seventies black leather Buffalo bag by Carlos Falchi. Or channel Carla Bruni-Sarkozy in head-to-toe dove grey Dior, a picture of Gallic charm and understated eroticism.

Always interpret fashion individually, with pieces picked out with care and assembled with a smattering of taste and savoir-faire. Buy clothes with attention to cut and detail that flatter and enhance your curves, items that will remain fabulous from season to season.

Recently, the British fashion designer Vivienne Westwood, known for her unconventional approach, declared that we should stop buying clothes for six months. *'If you engage with life, you will get a new set of values; get off the consumer treadmill and start to think – it is these great thinkers who will rescue the planet.'* This may seem a little radical, but through making more considered choices and paying slightly more for fewer, but better-quality clothes, you will play your part. Developing more of an eco-approach to fashion is the ultimate in sophisticated sustainability.

As fashion moves away from the throwaway to a collection of exquisite and considered purchases, clothes become invested with greater emotional meaning and memories, precious heirlooms to be handed down rather than disposed of after a weekend's wear. In buying well and combining the best of today with, say, the most exquisite vintage of the past, you will create a personalized wardrobe imbued with more meaning.

So, take a space-age perspex Chanel cuff or string of Bohemian glass beads sourced from the Parisian Marché aux Puces and mix it with classic couture in shades of cream and white. Find a little black dress that works for you and cover your shoulders with a fringed and beaded Art Deco wrap. Do Fifth Avenue fashion like Catherine Zeta Jones channelling Ava Gardner in a full-length mink (faux is less Cruella de Vil!), black stilettos, fly-eye shades and a chic chignon. Drape yourself in a Grecian-style wool jersey evening gown from neck to toe while remaining spectacularly sexy like Jennifer Aniston. In this way, vintage can mix with modern while modern has lasting appeal, mapping out a whole new autobiography.

A WARDROBE FOR THE *A-List*

Take heritage-modern as your style mantra. There are some classic pieces of fashion that every woman should own and they've all been worn by the most stylish of stars. The beauty is that you don't have to be a pre-pubescent model or a slouchy Sienna Miller type – they truly look better on glamorous grown-ups!

TAKE 1 *The Trench*

Once the perfect solution to a very British problem, the rain, but now a look that has gone global and is worn by glamorous grown-ups such as Michelle Pfeiffer, Demi Moore, Sharon Stone and Lauren Hutton (who wore a classic trench with a sexy twist in a shimmering metallic leopardskin print to Milan Fashion Week in 2009).

———————★———————

Your trench should be longer than any skirt underneath. The only exception is a pencil skirt under a mini-trench worn with heels. Jeans go with a trench like caviar and sour cream, so feel free to channel your inner Jackie O.

Wearing a classic trench saves both your inner psyche and your outer clothes and is thus an indispensable item for every grown-up's wardrobe. With its air of executive chic and ability to walk the tightrope between conservative and sexy, it suits the older woman. On someone young, it simply looks faux. Teenage fashion depends for a large part on showing off large areas of nubile flesh – leave that vulgarity to the young! Channel Kim Novak and wear your trench with a headscarf, fly-eye shades and lipstick – look, you're revealing nothing and you look drop dead gorgeous!

GROWN-UP GLAMOUR
Takes to the Trenches

★ **MARLENE DIETRICH IN MANPOWER** (1941) reveals the trench's mysterious side by wearing one in noir with matching heels.

★ **SOPHIA LOREN** does Italian-style trench in **THE KEY** (1958) and instantly explodes the myth that busty girls can't wear them.

★ In **VIVRE SA VIE** (1962) **ANNA KARINA** wears a trench coat with black heels and bare legs. OK, she plays a woman who descends into prostitution, but dammit, she looks good!

★ **MERYL STREEP** in **KRAMER VS. KRAMER** appeared to kick-start a trench revival in 1979, but Angie Dickinson's contribution in the *Police Woman* TV series should never be under-estimated.

★ In episode 12 of the cult classic Eighties mini-series **SINS, JOAN COLLINS** wears a camel Burberry trench with a black polo-neck sweater underneath, a leopardskin headscarf and red lipstick. You know it makes sense.

The Burberry trench, with its trademark check lining introduced in 1924, is the Rolls-Royce of waterproof raincoats. It was designed by Thomas Burberry for British Army officers in 1914 and made from cotton gabardine, which makes the coat waterproof, breathable, comfortable and supple. The company now make the same silhouettes in much more pliable materials, if that takes your fancy. All in all, this chic and classic outer envelope will be around forever.

─────── ★ ───────

Black trench coats need to be worn above the knee or you'll look like an off-duty policewoman or Keanu Reeves in *The Matrix*. Short girls should never wear red trench coats. Being mistaken for the murderous midget in the Seventies movie *Don't Look Now* is never a good look!

GETTING IT RIGHT

★ Although the trench has a belt, don't buckle it – just tie it at the waist like Kim Cattrall in *Sex and the City*. If you haven't got much of a waist and it feels too bulky, leave it open!

★ Make sure the epaulettes end at the shoulder seam and the button-centre vent doesn't pull open at the back when you fasten it, otherwise your bum will stick out like Max Wall!

Kim Cattrall shows how a woman in her fifties can ooze class and understated sexiness in a classic trench. Note the classic tied, rather than buckled, belt.

★ Do the double-breasted Burberry, not the single-breasted with the placket front or you'll resemble the placid wife of a right-wing politician.

★ You do not, repeat do not, have to buy a new one – there are lots of high street copies but steer clear of any attempting a Burberry-esque check lining. It will look too sad. Beware fake Burberry – clue: the stitching should be impeccable.

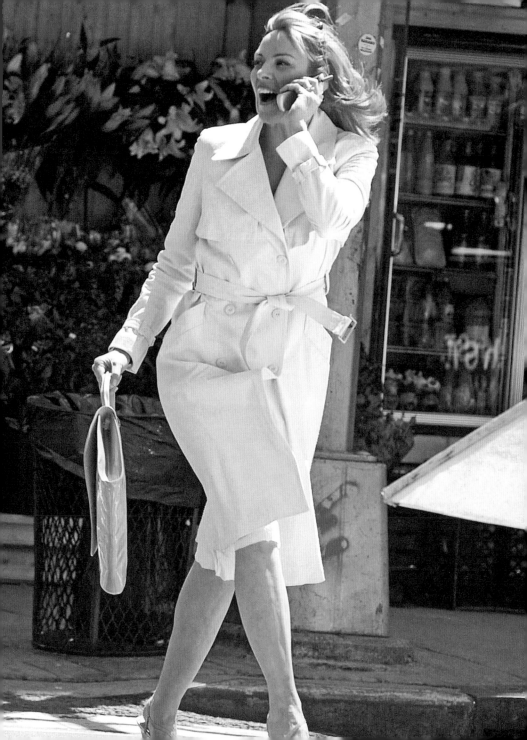

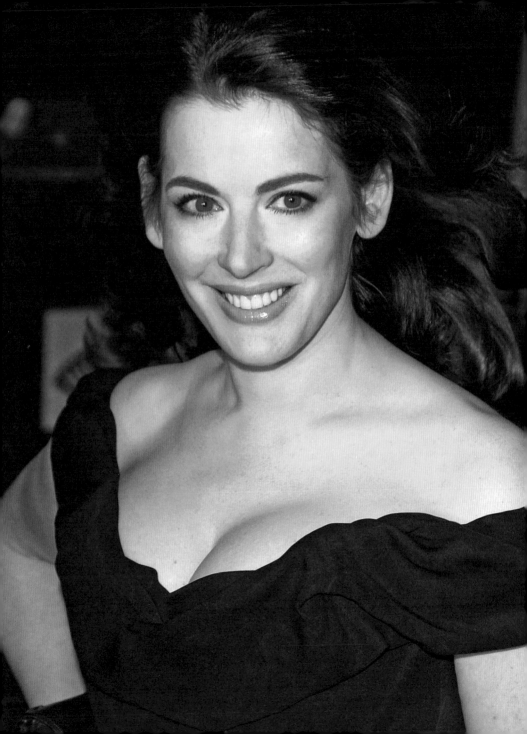

❋ ❋ ❋ ❋ ❋ ❋ ❋ ❋ ❋ ❋ ❋ ❋

TAKE 2 *The Little Black Dress*

When an older woman wears a LBD she is making an enduring style statement by placing herself in a roll call of the world's most compelling older women. Jackie O wore an LBD for both day and night, Marlene Dietrich wore them very well, and in 2010, Sophia Loren – at the age of 75 – recycled the same LBD to the Golden Globe Awards and a cocktail party in London a few months before. Who could blame her? It was black, form-fitting to show off her hour-glass curves to perfection, with a saucy sweetheart neckline and short, sheer, bead-studded sleeves to cover one of those little problem areas many of us have – the upper arms.

So, why does this look suit glamorous grown-ups best of all? Quite simply, the LBD is the essence of chic and the last word in sophistication, the black lines giving a silhouette both luxurious and austere in its graphic lines. In 1926, Coco Chanel invented this soignée look in response to the theatrical excess of couturier Paul Poiret. She recognized that bits of frippery might well suit the young, but the mystery and allure of the LBD requires someone with worldly wisdom to carry it off. As Coco once said, in a well-known criticism of her rival Paul Poiret, *'Scheherazade is easy. A little black dress is difficult.'*

Nigella Lawson in her trademark 'off the shoulder' LBD. Her love of this look is such that in 2009 she spent nearly £2,000 on identical dresses by designer Katya Wildman.

LBDS WORK BECAUSE:

★ They make glamorous grown-ups feel slimmer, a must when the passing of years can sometimes add a few extra pounds – so psychology is on your side!

★ The stripped-down style means you can add your own signature like a colour-popping scarf or a jangling charm bracelet. Sandra Bullock almost always wears an LBD on the red carpet and makes it her own with her choice of jewellery, whether it be huge gold hoop earrings or multi-strands of faux pearls.

★ As fashion designer Mary Quant put it in *Colour By Quant*, an LBD has: 'a chameleon sex appeal' that can be all things to all older women. *'It can be demure, as in the ubiquitous little black dress that clings with subtle suggestiveness to otherwise unsuspected curves. It can hit the heights of drama in black satin. Black is romantic in lace, voluptuous in velvet.'*

★ Glamorous grown-up Grace Coddington – the American *Vogue* visionary of fashion – is never out of an LBD and says, *'A little black dress never overpowers; it allows a woman to play a whole range of parts.'*

GETTING IT RIGHT

From high street to high-end boutique, LBDs are available at every price point in all the following styles. There's no need to break the bank!

HALTER-NECK – A style favoured by Halle Berry, who wore a knockout version with beaded python trim by Roberto Cavalli to the 2009 NAACP Image Awards. Halle showed us that the halter-neck is great for drawing attention to the cleavage and shoulders and takes emphasis away from heavier hips. You don't have to display your arms if you feel insecure about them – a simple shrug is always sweet. For evening, wear a black sequined dinner jacket insouciantly over the top.

⎯⎯⎯★⎯⎯⎯

Never wear a necklace with a halter and always choose a dress with adjustable neckties rather than fixed or you'll be left with a permanent stoop halfway through the day!

SLEEVELESS SHEATH DRESS – In 2007, Julia Roberts wore a sleeveless black shift with patent leather trim by Dolce & Gabbana accessorized with thick gold bangles to a film première. The sheath looks fabulous on lean, older women and has a sophistication that does not suit the young – ha! Its simple lines draw attention to the proportions of the body like no other, so those with a voluptuous or hourglass figure should avoid it. The perfect accompaniment to this *Breakfast at Tiffany's* classic is a pair of above-elbow length black evening gloves and pearls that draw a soft light to your skin and play down the outfit's solemnity. Don't do the cigarette holder and chignon, though – you'll veer perilously close to fancy-dress!

WRAP DRESS – Marisa Tomei wore the most amazing vintage Halston black silk wrap dress to the 2010 *Vanity Fair* Oscars party. This classic was actually invented by designer Diane von Furstenberg in 1974. It's cut to flatter your curves. If you're short of cash, Banana Republic does an elegant (and much cheaper) version! Vivienne Westwood wraps have great draping on the front for the bolder of belly, another awkward area for the older woman.

★

Wraps look good on the buxom of bosom, but grown-up girls need to be careful as the ties can become loose and this style of dress can fall away at the cleavage to reveal rather more flesh than anticipated. Solve the problem by wearing a sleeveless tee or black lace chemise underneath.

OFF THE SHOULDER – Designers Vivienne Westwood and Donna Karan are real enthusiasts for this look and understand what works for the older woman. Glamorous grown-ups have fantastic shoulders; it's a place where almost nothing can go wrong! You will be exposing flesh, but not uncomfortably so and the width at the top of the dress balances out the hips.

In 2009, voluptuous TV chef Nigella Lawson spent nearly £2,000 on 12 identical dresses by designer Katya Wildman, which bore a striking resemblance to the rest of the dresses in her wardrobe. Now there's a glamorous grown-up who has found her bombshell style! The Nigella dress is off the shoulder, an LBD type that definitely suits women with curves and not the young, who have yet to develop them!

SEVEN STEPS TO ELEGANCE
by Marlene Dietrich

★ Don't ever follow the latest trend, because in a short time you will look ridiculous.

★ Don't buy red, green or any other flamboyant colour dress.

★ A small wardrobe must consist of outfits you can wear again and again.

★ Don't believe the sales talk that you can have five dresses for the price of one.

★ Don't buy cheap materials, no matter how attractive the dress looks to you.

★ Don't say you can't afford a dress made of expensive materials. Save up for it.

★ While you're saving for that good black dress, on your next date wear a black sweater and skirt. Nothing wrong with that as long as you don't ruin the elegance of the outfit by overemphasis of the bosom.

'GEORGE CLOONEY IS
LIKE A CHANEL SUIT, HE'LL
NEVER GO OUT OF STYLE.'

CARRIE BRADSHAW IN *SEX AND THE CITY*

TAKE 3 *The Chanel Suit*

The ubiquitous Chanel suit – a collarless, braid-trimmed cardigan with matching skirt – is worn by glamorous grown-ups Penelope Cruz, Barbara Walters, Claudia Schiffer and Catherine Deneuve. In a mix of jersey and tweed, the Chanel suit dates from 1954 and was popularized by the divine Jackie Kennedy. The jacket is collarless with gilt buttons and the skirt is slim, but not overly so. Classic French chic makes the young look as if they're dressing up in mummy's clothes, while the older woman looks like she can take on the world!

GETTING IT RIGHT

★ You could go the whole Chanel route and accessorize with a black quilted chain and leather handbag, two-tone slingbacks and a camellia corsage, but it is a little Ivana Trump!

★ Broad of hip? Just wear the jacket with a knee-length skirt.

★ Faux Chanel is fine if you haven't got the funds – stores such as Marks & Spencer sell convincing high-street imitations.

★ The pale pink version suits every skin tone.

★ A real Chanel suit may be outrageously pricey, but it's the little details such as the weighted hem of the jacket that make authentic Chanel so luxe. This is a suit that will last forever and never date – as Chanel said: '*A fashion that goes out of fashion overnight is a distraction, not a fashion.*'

TAKE 4 *The White Shirt*

A memorable fashion moment was when Sharon Stone wore her husband's crisp white shirt to the 1998 Oscars, teaming it with a Vera Wang lavender silk skirt, so proving the white shirt works anywhere. A white shirt goes with practically everything! It freshens up the older women's complexion by throwing light up to the face – worldwide, it's also the greatest-ever hangover cure. What's not to like?

Once a bastion of male style, it's been a staple of women's wardrobes since the Eighties while today's designers are paying more attention to the details. If you want to see just how fantastic a white shirt can be, look up environmentalist-turned-designer Anne Fontaine (annefontaine.com), who has created two collections of an eye-popping 500 tailored shirts for women every year since 1993. This canny designer realized that a white shirt is fashion's blank canvas on which any amount of classic cool or frothy fantasy can be projected, fashioned out of cotton piqué, poplin or organdy.

GETTING IT RIGHT

★ Go for a darted semi-fitted or fitted one rather than a classic dress shirt, as they can make the most petite heroine look bulky. If a cardigan is worn over a classic, it can bunch up into a dowager's hump. Audrey Hepburn famously wore a man's white shirt tied at the back to show off her waist.

★ Shoulder seams should always line up with your natural shoulder and buttons must never pull across the front.

★ For the best fit, the bust-line darts of a fitted or semi-fitted shirt should always fall below the centre of the bust. When Jennifer Lopez wears a white shirt, the darts always fall below the bust to help give her shirt a tailored look.

★ You should be able to shoot your cuffs without them pulling away at the wrist.

★ Leave at least two, but properly three buttons open to reveal a hint of cleavage and a flattering line from face to embonpoint. Kate Hudson does this brilliantly, usually in Zac Posen (zacposen.com).

★ Lands End (landsend.co.uk) and Brooks Brothers (brooksbrothers.com) are good for a no-iron (yeess!), straight-collar classic. Elena Mirò (elenamiro.com) and Eskandar (eskandar.com) are superb for larger sizes and quirky styling. Try Ted Baker (tedbaker.com) for a little twist with your classic and Calvin Klein Petites (available at most department stores) for the exquisite miniatures among you. Avoid Thomas Pink because life's too short for ironing!

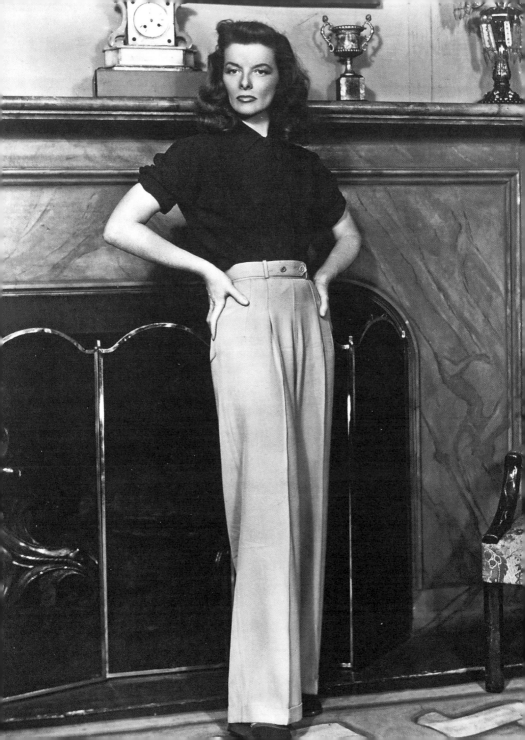

TAKE 5 *The Perfect Trousers*

Glamorous grown-up Katharine Hepburn knew that perfect trousers are wide enough to fall in a straight line from hip to floor and have a zip at the side, not the front. This shape seriously suits everybody. If you have any problems in the tummy area (and let's face it, most of us grown-up girls usually do), a fly front combined with a trouser that has a low rise will buckle over unflatteringly – this shape will not go in under your stomach, a problem with most other types of pants. You'll also avoid the dreaded muffin top.

——————★——————

Joseph trousers are cut for the tall and thin, so that's you sorted if you have skinny legs. Hobbs stock this style every season up to a British size 18 (American 14).

GETTING IT RIGHT

★ The key to finding this trouser shape in your size is, unfortunately, to try lots on. Getting the lie of the crotch right is crucial or you'll find yourself revealing a little too much information about your most private of areas. Different designers use different pattern blocks and so it's a process of trial and error to find the particular one for you, but when you've found it, your trouser problems are sorted for life!

★ This shape of trouser can be glammed up with wedges – Jan Jansen (janjansenshoes.com) do the most interesting, if you're prepared to ignore the 'art' shoes clearly worn only by textile lecturers who wish they were Virginia Woolf! Classic white or black plimsolls, or a pair of Converse trainers (sneakers) look cool as cucumber in summer.

Screen icon Katharine Hepburn shows off the perfect trouser shape for glamorous grown-ups with a side zip rather than a front fly.

✿ ✿ ✿ ✿ ✿ ✿ ✿ ✿ ✿ ✿ ✿ ✿

TAKE 6 *The Bias Cut Skirt*

Editor of American *Vogue* Anna Wintour always gets it right and she loves a bias cut skirt – New York Fashion Week usually sees her wearing one accessorized with a hip-length sable fur coat.

——— ★ ———

When you try the skirt on, it should not go under the butt and then flare out – this happens when the side seams are overly curved. If it does, you'll get an odd fishtail effect at the back, or look as if you've just been to the powder room and tucked your skirt into your knickers.

Because they are cut diagonally, bias cut garments have a very different look to ordinary clothes – even when the same basic pattern or shape is used, there's a real sexiness, delicacy and flow. For decades, Calvin Klein and Donna Karan have both favoured bias cut faille satins and slub silk in their collections, deluxe materials expertly cut to slide when the body moves.

GETTING IT RIGHT

★ The key is length: ankle-length is perfect for evening, otherwise it should hit the knee for the right 'flippy' effect. Anything between knee and ankle looks mumsy and if you combine with a droopy cardigan, 'Shazam!' instant celibacy!

★ If the skirt is too small and the seams are too curved, there'll be a jodhpur effect at the sides as the skirt rides up and your thighs will be revealed when you sit down.

★ If you have big calves, don't wear a short bias without opaque tights and boots. (Please, never, ever wear pointy-toed stretch boots either – vile, vile, vile!)

TAKE 7 *The Maxi Dress*

No matter what their age, weight or height, in summer or winter glamorous grown-ups can wear a maxi dress. They are not just for the young – in fact, they have an inverse effect, making older women look younger and vice versa. Heidi Klum, Eva Longoria and Sarah Jessica Parker all throw on a maxi dress for summer in the city.

Maxi dresses are multi-functional and the ultimate in comfort, yet incredibly fresh and fashion forward. They also hide a multitude of sins. Wear with a cropped cardigan, shades and an over-sized bag – très chic!

★

The myth is that short girls can't wear maxis. Rubbish, they look amazing! You just have to choose the right one. The material should be soft cotton or silk and avoid any kind of fussy embellishment. A scoop or strapless neckline will draw the line down and make your body appear longer – wear with wedge heels rather than flip-flops.

GETTING IT RIGHT

★ For winter, take one black maxi dress, team with cropped black leather jacket and biker boots. Go on, I dare you!

★ Voluptuous girls really suit an Empire line. Comedienne Dawn French never looked better than when parodying Catherine Zeta Jones in a black, bejewelled Empire-line maxi.

★ Never wear a belt with a maxi: it clutters up the silhouette. Don't combine tailoring with a maxi, either – it looks schizo.

★ Heels plus a maxi dress send it straight into Seventies dinner party territory.

TAKE 8 *The Cashmere Cardigan*

Knitted from the downy undercoat of the Kashmir goat, cashmere melts like butter on your skin. It clung in all the right places when worn by Jackie O and Grace Kelly with their triple strands of pearls. Today Sheryl Crow wears one with nothing underneath plus a pair of skinny jeans and Sigourney Weaver wears cashmere cardigans everywhere, thrown over wide-legged pants and evening dresses. Under-thirties need not apply, as this look suits the older woman best – it's the epitome of discreet elegance.

The cashmere cardigan was brought into evening wear in the 1950s by American designer Mainbocher, who was described by *Time Magazine* as *'the master of the throwaway: a little tweed jacket that suddenly turns out to be lined with sable, a simple something buttoned up to the neck that unbuttons – if you just happen to feel like it – to reveal a splash of Schlumberger or Verdura in emeralds and diamonds.'*

Mainbocher's embellished cashmere cardigans were first worn by style arbiters Gloria Vanderbilt, Babe Paley and Bunny Mellon and copied by thousands of women. Luckily, there are lots of beautiful beaded vintage cardigans. Look for details like mother of pearl buttons, braided and ribbon detail plus all sorts of little sequin gee-gaws. Every grown-up girl has the right to a cashmere cardigan – wear with a long evening skirt in shantung silk or a strappy silk slip dress.

GETTING IT RIGHT

★ Cashmere comes in different grades: the higher the grade, the better the cashmere. Your cardigan will be more expensive, but it will last longer and pill less. Similarly, the higher the ply, the weightier and more expensive it is.

★ Store your cashmere in one of the drawers in the freezer, then it won't get the moths and will pill less when worn.

★ The care label may read 'dry clean only', but cashmere aficionados believe handwashing a cashmere sweater makes it softer over time. Just be sure to use a baby shampoo or a mild detergent. Press out the excess water. Never wring the sweater. Lay it flat on a towel and reshape as it dries.

★ Avoid creating a line that runs down the middle by folding each side of the sweater inward by a third. Now smooth the arms down, and fold in half. Never, ever hang a wet cashmere sweater – the pull of gravity will distort its shape and create dimples in the shoulders where you put the pegs.

★ Buying vintage? Look out for the name Helen Bond Carruthers, who specialized in breathtakingly beautiful cropped and appliquéd cardigans in the 1950s that were worn by A-Listers like Elizabeth Taylor. The designer customized simple cashmere cardigans from Bergdorf Goodman with hand-embroidered appliqué cut from antique Chinese shawls. They were then lined in silk chiffon and the sleeves shortened to three-quarter length. The label is always in the grosgrain ribbon waistband.

'I WANT TO BE THE BEST-DRESSED WOMAN IN THE WORLD WITHOUT APPEARING TO BE THE BEST-DRESSED WOMAN IN THE WORLD.'

JACKIE O

Jackie O used sunglasses to ward off unwanted attention and disguise her wide set eyes. She always made sure her sunglasses were big enough to cover one third of her face.

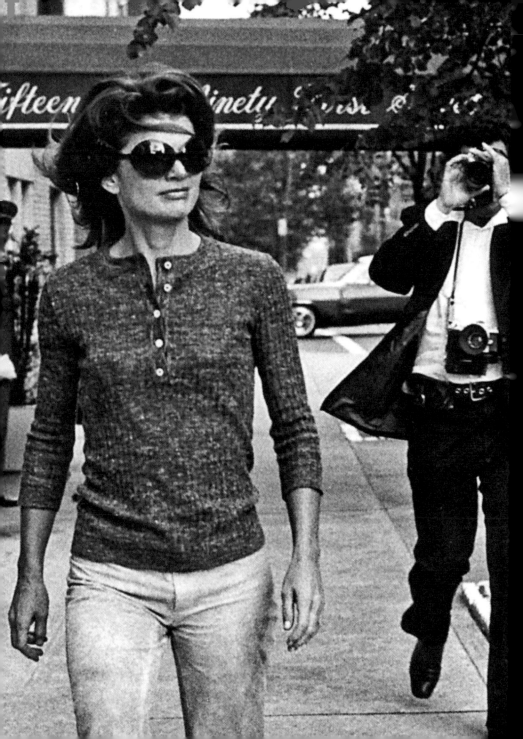

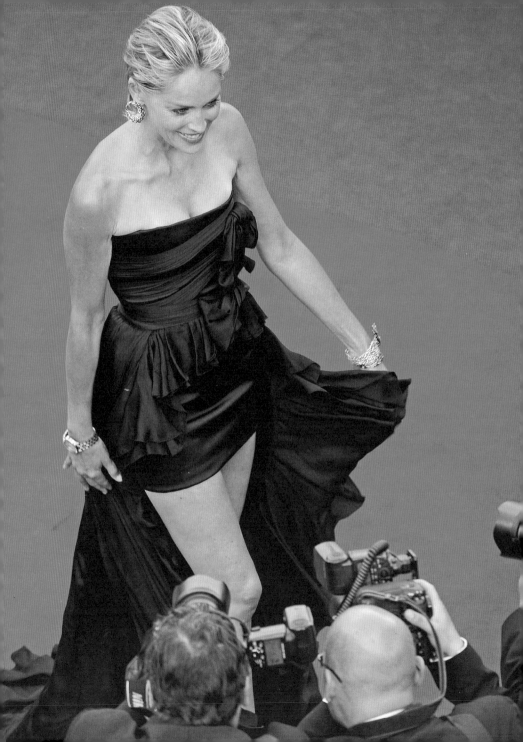

So **LAST YEAR...**

'YOU CAN'T WEAR A MINISKIRT OVER THE AGE OF 28'

★ It's not a question of age for miniskirts, more whether or not you have the legs for it. The popular fallacy is that you have to stop wearing a mini after 28 – rubbish! As the American designer Bill Blass once said, 'The legs are the last to go!'

★ Obviously extreme minis are out or you'll look like a hooker, but above the knee is fine so long as you wear opaque tights in black, navy, plum or dark jewel tones.

★ In 2009, Sharon Stone wore a thigh-skimming black silk Balmain micromini to a film première in Cannes at the age of 51 and looked fabulous! (If anyone protests, say it's not the skirt that's too short, it's your legs that are too long!)

★ Is there a cut-off point? Well, Jerry Hall's teenage daughter banned her mother from wearing them when she hit 50. Georgia May Jagger says: 'I did take all her miniskirts. I told her one night that her skirt was too short – she came down the stairs and I was like, "God, Mum, you are 50!"' We say: Jerry, you need to move the kids out and the minis back in!

NEVER...

★ Show bare knees, unless on the French Riviera in the height of summer. If Brigitte Bardot is still doing it, so can you!

★ Have a matching jacket or you'll look like a pastel power-suited Alexis Colby.

★ Wear with high heels – too Phuket lady boy!

Sharon Stone wows Cannes in 2009 in a Balmain LBD. She may be able to get away with bare legs in a micro mini but on us mere mortals it's a little unforgiving.

'LEOPARD PRINT WILL MAKE YOU LOOK CHEAP'

★ Think fashion panache, not barmaid trash! Contemporary designers such as Alber Elbaz at Lanvin have totally re-invented the leopard look, and Stephen Sprouse's signature print scarves in several different colourways (the navy/pink is lush!) are a seasonal staple at Louis Vuitton (see louisvuitton. com for stockists).

★ A vintage leopard print swing coat looks amazing over a black polo neck and pencil skirt combo at any age and is super-glam over a black cocktail dress at night.

★ Always remember that leopard does not automatically have to mean the traditional markings of black and tan, although Dolce & Gabbana are always masters at re-creating that Fifties Italian starlet look – perfect for any heroine happy to channel her inner Gina Lollobrigida!

★ Pink and grey, or camouflage colours are a sophisticated take on an old fashion favourite and can be found at Left Bank label Isabel Marant (isabelmarant.tm.fr), printed on flirty chiffon and silk tea dresses, as worn by Rachel Weisz. Claudia Schiffer wore a stunning green and black print mini to a London Fashion Week dinner in 2009, breaking two taboos at once (NB: she also wore black opaque tights).

★ If your disposition is too delicate for full-on leopard, opt for a bag instead. As far as I am concerned, the best is the Mulberry Piccadilly in Smudged Leopard, but it has to be putty (mulberry.com). The classic suede-lined Bayswater, complete with its trademark postman's lock, comes in cool coral, too. Now, where did I put my Amex?

NEVER...

★ Wear more than one type of leopard print at once – it's way too 'Working Girl' (and I don't mean Melanie Griffith!).

★ Wear above-ankle leopard boots or you'll look brassy.

★ Pick winklepicker stilettos in leopard unless you want to be labelled an HRT poisoned 'cougar' and that's always a difficult label to shake off. OK, it's a jungle out there, but you don't want to be seen to be so obviously stalking your prey!

★ There's no 'fun' in fun fur, whether leopard or not – dressing 'cheerfully' is the first stop on a fast train to senility.

★ If you don't feel daring enough to wear leopard print, live with it! Jackie O covered the White House furniture with leopard throws.

RULES *Definitely* SET IN STONE

ABSOLUTELY NO, NADA, NIET...

★ Crop tops, tattoos or intimate piercing unless you're trying to blend in at an Everglades trailer park.

★ Chiffon sleeves – they make any arms look fat!

★ Black leather trousers – you're not Suzi Quatro and the kids will blanch!

★ High-waisted 'mummy' jeans occasionally sported by (gulp, dare I say it?) Joan Collins.

★ Gypsy skirts and Cuban-heeled cowboy boots – you will immediately take on the mantle of the Sixties rock chick suspended in aspic, especially if combined with long, flicky blonde hair. But if you want to open a cat sanctuary and spend your days earnestly tendering to ginger toms while listening to Fleetwood Mac's Tusk, go right ahead.

★ Stonewashed denim – if you wore it first time around, shame on you! Why suffer the same trauma (and Tiffany singles) again?

★ 'Girlie' fashion. Unfortunately any hint of frilly pink, puffed sleeves or ra-ra will make you look like Grayson Perry.

★ Elasticized waists – unless you live in a gated community.

★ Patchwork: please stash it away with your juggling balls – you're no longer a member of Spiral Tribe.

MAINBOCHER'S
Fashion Mantras

★ 'To be well turned out, a woman should turn her thoughts in.'

★ 'I have never known a really chic woman whose appearance was not, in large part, an outward reflection of her inner self.'

★ 'I don't want my clothes to make a woman look desperate for attention; I do want them to add to her chic and not make her look smarty smart.'

WHERE TO SHOP FOR
Vintage Chic

Chart your own fashion path by buying vintage. Just about anyone can walk down the high street and obtain the latest looks off the rail, but there's always the danger that you might find yourself reaching for the same top in mirror image! If you become a connoisseur of vintage chic, not only will your style be much more individual style, but you'll also compile a wardrobe of rich heritage pieces that can be passed down from this generation to the next.

Most cities have a gem of a vintage store tucked away and here's our guide to some of the finest:

★ **AMSTERDAM: LADY DAY**
Haartenstrat 9
(theninestreets.com/ladyday.html)
Two floors of quality vintage clothing, from the 1950s–80s.

★ **BARCELONA: THE RIERA BAIXA**
Tiny street, with a plethora of second-hand and vintage stores that seem to open and close almost overnight.

★ **BERLIN: MODEMARKT FREESTYLE**
Bergmannstrasse 102, Kreuzeberg
One for your secret address book: a tremendous selection of fashion from most eras.

★ **COPENHAGEN: WETTERGREN & GRAUMANN,** *Laederstraede 5 1201*
Expensive and exclusive!

★ **HELSINKI: PLAY IT AGAIN SAM**
Rauhankatu 2, 00170
Tailored suits and day dresses, 1940s–70s.

★ **LISBON: A OUTRA FACE DA LUA**
22 Rua da Assunção
(aoutrafacedalua.com)
Lovely Twenties finds, plus quirky reworked vintage-modern pieces.

★ **LONDON: VINTAGE MODES AT GRAY'S ANTIQUES**, *Davies Street, W1 (graysantiques.com)*
A treasure trove of past styles, Kate Moss is a frequent visitor.

★ **MADRID: HOLALA**, *7 Calle del Paz*
Smack-bang in the stylish shopping district of Malsana.

★ **MILAN: L'ARMADIO DI LAURA** *Via Voghera, 25 (armadiodilaura.it)*
Exclusive and elegant, this shop is tucked away in a tiny courtyard behind huge wooden doors.

★ **NEW YORK: KENI-VALENTI RETRO-COUTURE**, *155 West 29th Street (kenivalenti.com)*
The 'King of Vintage' has a jaw-dropping collection in this swanky showroom.

★ **OSLO: TRABANT CLOTHING COMPANY**, *Markvelen 56 (trabantclothing.com)*
Slick little store featuring clothing from 1950–80.

★ **PARIS: MARCHE AUX PUCES DE SAINT-OUEN**, *Porte de Clignancourt, 75018 (les-puces.com)*
The largest fleamarket in Paris is full of vintage finds, from couture to tat, especially the Marché Vernaison.

★ **STOCKHOLM: LISA LARSSON** *Bondegatan 48 (lisalarssonsecondhand.com)*
Tiny, but well established shop – the focus of vintage enthusiasts for more than 20 years.

★ **TOKYO: SWIPE** *5-32-13 Daizawa, Setagaya-ku*
Plethora of Eighties clothes at reasonable prices.

★ **VIENNA: BOCCA LUPO** *Landskrongasse 1-3*
Specializes in high-end Louis Vuitton, Hermès and Chanel.

★ **ZURICH: LUX PLUS**, *Ankerstrasse 24*
Beautifully curated vintage fashion, including folksy, embroidered Swiss blouses.

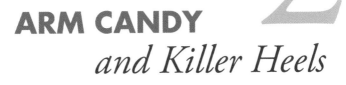

ARM CANDY
and Killer Heels

What sacrifices would you have to make to afford Miu Miu's gorgeous 'Coffer' bag – all butter-soft leather, ruches and gold hardware, and a hefty price to boot? If you ate beans on toast for a month, could you stretch to Marc Jacobs' delicious plum metallic 'Mariah'? Such 'It' bags have become the ultimate twenty-first century object of desire, not just for supermodels and celebrities but for girls of all ages and incomes, from all walks of life. And that's just the problem: modern 'It' bags have become the mark not of those with taste, but of the shopaholic with her wallet full of maxed-out credit cards and a lust for the over-designed.

So many seasonal bags are being churned out that good design has all but disappeared. Ergonomics have fallen by the wayside as huge chain-wrapped totes spell dominatrix dungeon rather than a trip to the supermarket, while massive padlocks make bags so unbalanced they need a prop. Glamorous grown-ups should seize the moment and show that a literate understanding of designers, shapes and brands is of necessity when displaying your fashion cred.

So, don't make like a WAG and grab the nearest 'Stam' – bags are too important for that. As Carrie says in *Sex and the City*, 'I'm thinking balls are to men what purses are to women. It's just a little bag, but we feel naked in public without it.'

Be a BAG LADY

Glamorous grown-ups know that it's best to fix on a classic bag because real ones hold their value well, unlike the seasonal 'It'. You don't have to buy brand new either – reputable dress agencies always have a good range or you can track one down on eBay or Trade Me. It is a bit of a minefield out there, so if you have a bit more dash than cash or maybe you don't trust the internet auction sites, opt for a high-street lookalike instead.

Marnie Fogg, author of *Vintage Handbags* and an expert in her field, has the following advice for spotting a counterfeit vintage handbag: 'There is a fine line between an homage to a designer handbag and a straightforward fake or "knock-off". An homage is an inevitable effect of the trickle-down of ideas, what is illegal is imitating the registered trademark. The duck emblem on the Dooney & Bourke handbags has often been illegally pirated, as has the LV symbol on Louis Vuitton bags. Logo-patterned bags of plastic coated canvas are very easy to copy. Consult some of the many on-line sites that give very detailed information and provide contrasting images of both real and fake handbags. mypoupette.com is an American website, which for a fee will check the authenticity of a designer bag.'

GET *Real*

MARNIE FOGG SAYS 1 Know what the bag should look like by checking online designer sales sites and if possible, genuine handbags in designer boutiques.

2 Research the elements that make up the bag: what should it be lined in? Should it have feet? What does the base of the bag look like? Is there a d-ring inside? If so, where? Does it have a date code?

3 Examine the stitching. This should be very even and regular, with the same number of stitches found in similar locations on other bags in the series. For example, the leather tab that the handle attaches onto on any size Vuitton monogram Speedy bag will always have five regular, even stitches across the top.

4 Big brands do not sell seconds – these can only be purchased from registered outlets.

5 Some brands provide details that help authenticate the bag – for example, for the last 20 years Hermès have included discreet embossed stamps inside their bags to denote when the bag was made and by whom. Louis Vuitton uses a production code inside its bags for the same purpose.

6 Anything can be faked. Counterfeiters not only fake bags, but also fake the provenance details. These include receipts, boxes and even dust bags.

Jane Fonda with one-time husband Roger Vadim in Paris, toting a classic black lambskin quilted Chanel bag and stiletto heeled sling-backs. The result? Total Gallic glamour!

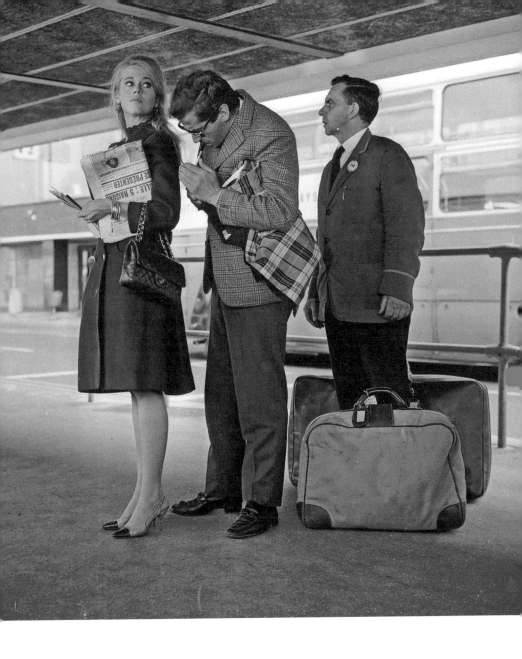

BAGS *of Style*

The following are some of the best examples of heritage-modern – great bags that work today and won't date. Once you know each one's stats you can either buy the original new or vintage, or source a convincing alternative.

────── ★ ──────

If the authenticity number is 9395451, do not buy! This number is used on lots of fake Chanel. Look closely at the zip – it should have 'Chanel' engraved on it in letters at least 1mm (0.03 in) thick. The raised double-'C' logo in the quilting should be perfectly stitched and the width of the letter consistent. You have a right to be suspicious of extremely low-priced bags, too.

CHANEL '2.55'

Coco's classic '2.55', or 'classic flap bag' as it is referred to in-store, made its first appearance in 1955 and was named after its month and year of birth. You know what it looks like – black diamond quilted lambskin (inspired by jockey's outfits), a long gilt chain strap interlaced with black hide (to free up your hands) and discreet gilt hardware, which includes the double-'C' lock.

PLUS The small and medium size bags have a double flap closure with a secret pocket.

MINUS Oh, purlease! There aren't any. But if you plan to use your '2.55' frequently, go for the grainier Caviar leather version as the soft lambskin can scuff.

HIGH STREET Find a convincing homage in chains like Marks & Spencer. Each season ASOS (asos.com) does a Chanel '2.55'-type bag with woven chain and gold clasp. To try before you buy, go to bagborroworsteal.com or fashionhire.co.uk

SPOTTING A FAKE Always ask for the authenticity number.

FENDI *'Baguette'*

'I'm homeless! I'll be a bag lady. A Fendi bag lady, but a bag lady!' says Carrie Bradshaw. Fendi had a starring role in the *Sex and the City* series! The 'Baguette' is so-called because it is carried under the arm like a loaf of bread. One of the most successful bags of all time, it gained its status as folk costume for the super-rich when clutched under the arms of grown-up girls Madonna, Kate Hudson and Naomi Campbell.

———————★———————

Accessories guru Silvia Venturini has produced over 1,000 different designs for the 'Baguette' in more than 600 choices of luxurious materials (the black leather sequin-sprayed one is particularly gorge). Once a style has sold out, it's never repeated.

PLUS A clever interpretation of the idea of a bag as an exquisite one-off objet d'art. You'll probably never meet someone else with the same one. Yet its clasp – an interlocked double-'F' logo – makes it instantly recognizable.

MINUS The size of it. One well-known fashion editor had to carry a shopping bag to supplement the Baguette's lack of storage space. She claimed she was making an ironic gesture.

HIGH STREET The high street has the equivalent shape, (basically a soft luxe clutch with a short shoulder strap) and Accessorize do lovely, reasonably priced versions (monsoon.co.uk). To hire inexpensively for a week, visit handbaghirehq.

SPOTTING A FAKE If there is any plastic on it, then it's a fake. Straps should be leather, as should the back of the buckle. The buckle must be perfectly square; it should feel heavy and have 'Fendi' engraved on the sides. Real Fendis have a silk or satin jacquard lining with 'Fendi' woven in throughout.

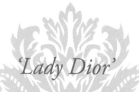

'Lady Dior'

Dior hit gold in 1994 when Diana, Princess of Wales, began carrying its square black crocodile double-handled tote with dangling charms that spelt out the Dior logo. This bag also comes in quilted leather and suede. Lady Diors have been spotted on the arms of glamorous grown-ups Charlize Theron, Penelope Cruz and Dita Von Teese. Fashion writer Mimi Spencer called it 'the visual equivalent of a yapping Chihuahua'.

———— ★ ————

'Made in France' on the interior tag means that it's a fake. Authentic Lady Diors have 'Made in Italy' on the back of the interior tag.

PLUS The epitome of French chic and a less obvious choice than the Chanel 2.55. Prices vary depending on whether you choose leather (still pricy, but more reasonable) or the croc version (you'll really need to shell out).

MINUS Can look a bit Sloane Ranger, if worn with a suit.

HIGH STREET The Jaeger Patent Dog Tooth Quilt Tote (jaeger.com) has the same feel and is a steal in comparison! To hire for a reasonable price per week, go to handbaghirehq.co.uk.

SPOTTING A FAKE The charms that dangle from the bag should all be in capital letters with the 'O' over-sized. Rings used to attach the handles to the bag should be stamped 'CD'. Inside the bag, the tag is usually of the same leather and reads 'Christian Dior Paris'. When lifted up, it should reveal a serial number made up of letters and numbers on the reverse side.

MCQUEEN *'Novak'*

Launched in 2005, the 'Novak' bag was named after Kim Novak, the legendary blonde who starred in Hitchcock's psychological thriller *Vertigo* (1958). Alexander McQueen took her structured Fifties look as inspiration for a deliberately 'uptight' bag in shiny Nappa stain-proof leather that blew all the slouchy Chloes out of the water.

PLUS Makes the YSL 'Muse' look positively adolescent. Price depends on size and choice of skin.

MINUS The serious mash-up of business and fetish can make grown men shrivel!

HIGH STREET A good structured bag will always be more expensive than something slouchy. Osprey of London's 'Polished Croc Grab' bag (ospreylondon.com) is beautiful, but pricey. A cheaper alternative is the Ri2K Ariel Grab Handbag in black. Both are available at John Lewis (johnlewis.com).

SPOTTING A FAKE It's relatively easy to spot the real thing because the high level of craftsmanship, precise stitching and attention to detail in the original 'Novak' are extraordinary – it's impossible to successfully fake. If the stitching is in any way wrong, swerve it!

FALCHI *'Buffalo'*

In 1974, Carlos Falchi created a truly inspired handbag – the 'Buffalo', a cross between a handbag and a duffel bag. This bag is seriously sexy and comes in an organic folded shape whose deep creases of black leather seem to mimic the hidden folds of the female body – ooh la la! Designer Carlos Falchi has been around for decades and is seriously ripe for a revival; his signature use of patchwork python skin is beyond belief! Cher carried one in the Seventies and now it's the turn of Eva Longoria, Marisa Tomei and Susan Sarandon. This could be the one for Chloe Sevigny, who once said, 'Too many bags flaunt huge labels. I prefer a more discreet look.'

PLUS Invites a suggestive glance and a sly touch.

MINUS You might have pervs committing frottage on your bag on a crowded bus!

HIGH STREET You'll never get an exact 'Buffalo' shape but the slouchy Hobo styles ape the orginal Falchi. Dorothy Perkins (dorothyperkins.com) always has a reasonably priced imitation black hobo, but why bother? Go to eBay, it's the place for Falchi and fantastic vintage Buffalos at low prices.

SPOTTING A FAKE Woo hoo! Haven't found one yet.

Jennifer Aniston has a icon of bag design casually slung across her shoulder – the Falchi Buffalo bag in camel. It comes in a myriad of colour-ways and sizes.

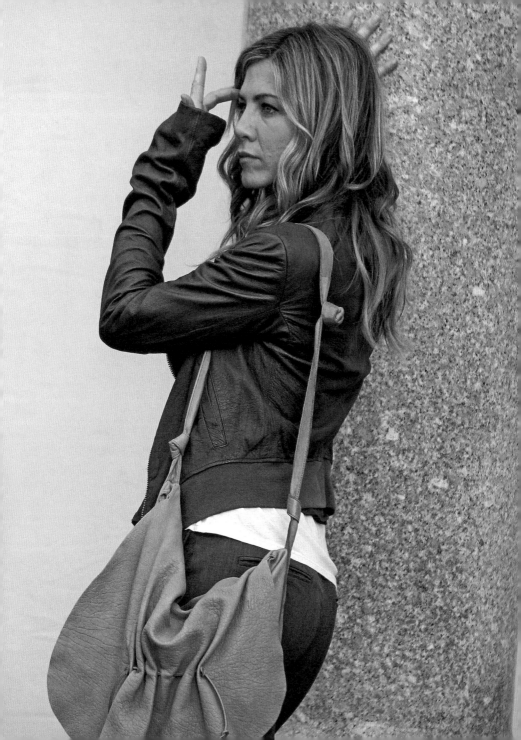

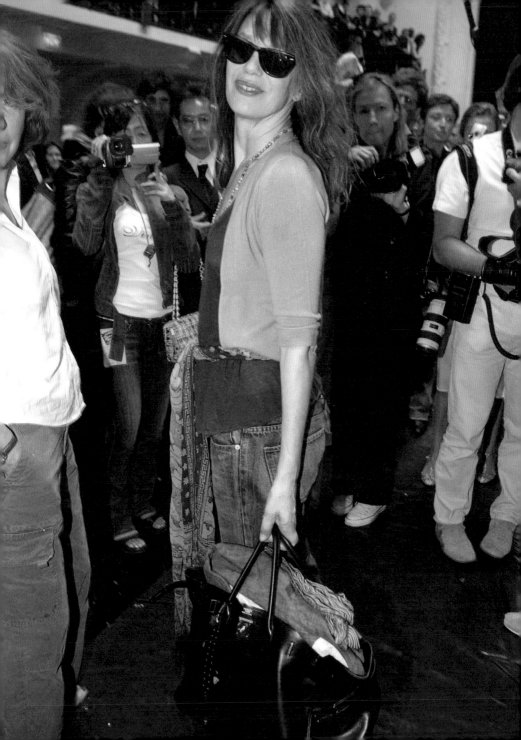

It's All in the **NAME**

The ultimate accolade is to have a designer bag named after you. Oh, mama – you've made it!

Gucci 'Jackie O'

Originally called the 'Constance' when first spotted on the arm of the elegant Jacqueline Kennedy Onassis. So many women asked for the 'Jackie' that Gucci jumped at the chance of a re-name. This lovely, double-strapped shoulder bag has a distinctive 'H' clasp.

Marc Jacobs 'Siouxsie'

Named after high priestess of punk Siouxsie Sioux as part of the 'Sweet Punk' line that includes the 'Debbie', after Debbie Harry. It's a supple, black leather studded bag but to me, it looks a little Camden Goth for the price tag. And it's lined in canvas for goodness sake!

Luella 'Joni'

Folky hippie deluxe, this gorgeous red leather studded bag with trademark Luella leather heart charms on the zip pull was named after singer Joni Mitchell.

Gucci 'Bardot'

Heroine of chic Brigitte Bardot scored this in the Sixties. With its monogrammed jacquard outer, single strap and leather trim, it still looks good 50 years on.

Jane Birkin with her namesake bag by Hermès. It travels with her everywhere and is customized with stickers and slogans drawing attention to her campaign for human rights.

Hermès 'Birkin'

In 1984, singer Jane Birkin sat next to Hermès president Jean-Louis Dumas with an overflowing, beaten-up straw bag. Asked to describe her dream arm candy, she came up with leather with a large opening – essentially a posh tote. Fast forward and Victoria Beckham has a Himalayan studded diamond version. Et Birkin? *'I love my Birkin bag, but I lug so much stuff around in it I believe it is part of the reason I have tendonitis,'* she revealed.

And just to show the youth of today don't appreciate a decent bag, actress Kelly Brook made the following confession about her Birkin in 2010: *'I never thought I'd spend that much on a bag, but I use it all the time. Although I was quite drunk on a night out and ended up being sick in it! But hey, better in there than in the cab, right?'*

Tod's 'D' Bag

Named after Princess Diana, who was regularly papped toting one, Tod's 'D' Bauletto handbag was launched in 1997 by designer Diego della Valle. It's a luxe-looking smooth calfskin bag with a distinctive roll top handle, zipper and gold-tone hardware. Its low key looks, discretion and absence of overt logos whisper a regal chic that only those 'in the know' will get and now you're in the know! Seen more recently on the arm of Nicole Kidman and Diane Kruger, it's not *too* fashion – the handbag incarnation of grown-up glamour.

'I HAVE A COUPLE OF GUCCI BAGS FROM WHEN TOM FORD WAS THERE. I LIKE TOD'S, I HAVE A MULBERRY PICCADILLY BAG AND I HAVE A GREAT BIG LOUIS VUITTON TOTE, BUT MY FAVOURITE BAG IS AN OLD WICKER PICNIC BASKET. IT WAS WOVEN BY NATIVE AMERICANS, AND I CARRY IT ALL SUMMER. EVERYONE THINKS I'VE BROUGHT MY OWN FOOD.'

MARIE HELVIN

If the Shoe FITS...

It's been estimated that most of us walk around 185,074 kilometres (115,000 miles) during our lifetime – although the figure will be considerably less for me if they keep running *Dynasty* back-to-back on UK TV! That means our poor tootsies are crammed into shoes for up to 16 hours per day.

The vacillation of fashionable footwear styles means that as we get older, our feet tend to wear out more quickly than men's, so it's vital to find the right fit. As glamorous grown-up Bette Midler says, 'Give a girl the correct footwear and she can conquer the world.' Just follow the tips below:

★ The right shoe size will help posture and back twinges.

★ You should be able to wriggle your toes in your shoes.

★ Never walk outside in new shoes – break 'em in at home!

★ Other than Havaianas worn strictly on the beach, avoid plastic shoes altogether.

★ As you get more grown-up, so too should your shoes. Age and weight gain mean your feet can change size like Cameron Diaz does boyfriends, so have your feet measured at least once a year.

★ Most of us have one foot bigger than the other – always fit to the larger foot and wear a padded insole in the other shoe so they match up.

Grown-Up **HEEL SHAPES**

Cone

Pure power Eighties, recently enjoying a revival and most associated with Manolo Blahnik and Maud Frizon. Cones are much easier to walk in than the stiletto and a shape that can be worn from day to night if you don't go too high. Diane Kruger wore a fab pair of strappy tan Lanvin cone heels plus platform soles to a Chanel party in Cannes (net-a-porter.com always has a good selection of the latest Lanvin).

Kitten

Invented in the Fifties as a form of starter heel for budding stiletto wearers, then combined with a pointed toe in the early Sixties, as worn by Brigitte Bardot. The heel must be less than 5cm (2in) high to qualify as kitten, but be careful: the height tends to foreshorten the calf and make the foot look bigger.

Despite the name, kittens have an edge of seriousness about them that means that they are a perennial favourite of the politician's wife (viz. Michelle Obama who buys her Jimmy Choos in three heights of heel, so she can move down over the day when they begin to pinch). They're a strategic shape for the woman who wants to remain heel-shod while not towering over her shorter consort (see Carla Bruni, Princess Diana). A little twee for my taste, LK Bennett has been dubbed Queen of the Kitten Heel (lkbennett.com).

Stiletto

This high heel has a metal spigot running inside the middle to give strength to its needle taper. A precision-engineered global phenomenon since it was first invented in the 1950s and most associated with designers Roger Vivier (rogervivier. com) and Christian Louboutin (christianlouboutin.com). The penetrating heel causes disturbance wherever it roams, with the click-click of its killer point causing hearts to race and those with hardwood floors to shudder.

The ultimate badge of status, authority and sex appeal for grown-up girls, it requires sexual maturity to deal with the commotion it causes. As worn by Grace Kelly, Sarah Jessica Parker ('As a short person – I'm 5'4" – I count on a nice heel'), Marilyn Monroe, Charlize Theron, Victoria Beckham, Jerry Hall, Anna Wintour – ach, just about every glamorous grown-up!

Screen diva Rita Hayworth in stiletto-heeled mules by David Evins. The Hollywood designer's shoes cut with a décolleté front in the 1940s were the first examples of 'toe cleavage'.

These heels do hurt, though, and as glamorous grown-ups, must we suffer the pain? At the 2008 Academy Awards, Renée Zellweger looked fabulous on the red carpet in her shimmering silver Carolina Herrera gown and Christian Louboutin stilettos but as the evening wore on, it seems she wished she'd gone for something a little more comfortable. After presenting an award, Renée was spotted backstage with her silver Louboutins slung over her shoulder. Johnny Depp approached and said, *'I like your shoes.'* *Renée shot back with a grimace: 'Thanks, man. I used to like them!'*

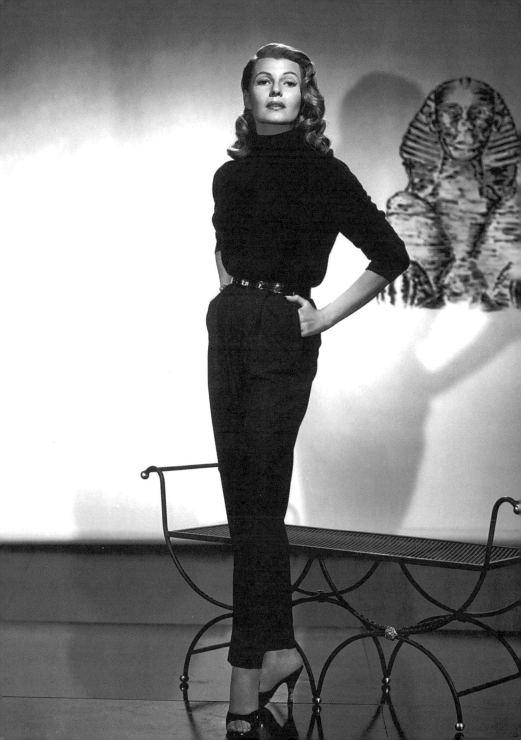

Wedge

Invented by Salvatore Ferragamo during the 1940s in response to the restrictions of war, when the steel used for shoe arches was in short supply, and then revived by Terry de Havilland in the 1970s and 2000s. Basically the space between the sole and the heel is filled in to support the foot, which is pretty darn perfect for giving height plus stability for glamorous grown-ups, as you are always balanced. Carmen Miranda, aka the Brazilian Bombshell, had an extensive wedge collection that, together with her towering tutti-frutti turbans, maximized her five-foot frame. Voluptuous girls should seek solace in a pair of wedges for evening – with my rather over-flowing hourglass shape, I always feel a little 'pig on stilts' in spikes.

As worn by glamorous grown-ups Eva Longoria, Jennifer Aniston and star of stage and screen Emma Thompson, who admits such a lust for shoes that she has to hide them from fellow actor husband, Greg Wise: '*He says, "Please don't tell me there's another pair of shoes coming into the house," so I hide them or scuff them so they don't look new, or pretend they cost 75p in a charity shop.*'

Love 'EM!

'I was born in high heels and I've worn them
ever since.'
HELENA CHRISTENSEN

'When I wear high heels I have a great vocabulary
and I speak in paragraphs. I'm more eloquent.
I plan to wear them more often.'
MEG RYAN

Loathe 'EM!

'I used to wear heels because I wanted to show people
I wasn't ashamed of being tall. But I don't wear them
any more because you don't have to wear heels to be
beautiful. I can't even remember the last time I wore
heels.'
ELLE MACPHERSON

'If I went out in killer heels and full make-up,
blow-dry, the whole thing – anyone dressed up like
that could be intimidating to men and women, really.
It's so, look at me. Do you know what I mean?'
RACHEL WEISZ

SHARING THE SPOTLIGHT:
Shoes on Screen

★ **MATA HARI** (1931) Greta Garbo appears dressed head-to-toe in gold lamé, including tight gold leggings and a pair of divine metallic boots by celebrated Hollywood costume designer Adrian. This was the look that inspired the bright gold toga dress that Marc Jacobs designed for Kate Moss's appearance at the Metropolitan Museum of Art's 2009 Costume Institute Gala. Moss was let down by the Stephen Jones shower cap and cheap-looking gold 'Tribute 2' heels by YSL, though. Didn't anyone have an Edit button?

★ **DOUBLE INDEMNITY** (1944) The slutty shoes, including the flash of naughty marabou mules outside the bedroom, worn by Barbara Stanwyck's Phyllis Dietrichson in this classic film noir should have warned off Fred MacMurray right from the start. But it's her ankle bracelet and pumps with the pouffes of tulle on the toes that really sow the seeds of Fred's downfall.

★ **THE SEVEN YEAR ITCH** (1955) Marilyn Monroe's white leather slingback Ferragamo stilettos are the ultimate in va va voom, but they're closely followed by her scarlet satin rhinestone-encrusted heels in *Gentlemen Prefer Blondes* (1953), later sold at Christies New York in 1999 for a cool $42,000.

★ **BELLE DE JOUR** (1967) Catherine Deneuve wears buckled pilgrim pumps by Roger Vivier and kickstarts a global fashion trend that included Marlene Dietrich and Jackie O. Today the Vivier label includes a pair of 'Belle' Vivier in every collection, updated by creative director Bruno Frisoni and in a range of searing colours (rogervivier.com).

★ **GILDA** (1946) Iconic Hollywood shoe designer David Evins created platform-heeled black satin slingbacks with ankle straps for Rita Hayworth. They are worn in the phenomenal opening striptease scene with a strapless black satin cocktail dress. Purrr-fect!

★ **FUNNY FACE** (1957) Salesgirl in a Greenwich bookstore by day, beatnik by night, a gamine Audrey Hepburn wears a black wool sweater, black Capri pants, white socks and flats in this fashion-focused movie. Hepburn was reputedly concerned about how such Left-Bank chic would work on screen, particularly the white socks that director Stanley Donen forced her to wear – she was convinced they would draw attention to her large feet. But Donen refused to capitulate to her demands, feeling that white socks would break up the dramatic all-black silhouette and pick out the steps she was making during an important freeform jazz-dance sequence. After the release, the star sent an apologetic note, 'You were right about the socks. Love, Audrey.' Offscreen, Hepburn wore black suede flats by Ferragamo with a low oval heel and shell sole based on the Native American opanke or moccasin.

Sophia Loren **TALKS SHOES**

'For many women, myself included, buying a pair of shoes is like a brief, sad love affair – the desire, the satisfaction, the disillusionment, the pain, all condensed in one afternoon. There is a more sinister aspect to uncomfortable shoes which I once heard a cynic express this way: "Yes, they are beautiful, those shoes, but notice how cruel. The young girl starts out in shoes like delicate canoes, but ends her life in ocean liners."

'This is a sad fact of life if you regularly sacrifice comfort for fashion where your feet are concerned. Eventually your poor feet will be tormented into corns and calluses and bunions and then you will be forced to wear ocean liners in order to walk. Those words stuck with me and even though I have dozens of pairs of beautiful shoes I wear the same ones all the time – the few pairs that are really comfortable and fit well.'

BOOTY *Call*

Glamorous grown-ups know that boots are subtly sexy, employing an under-rated eroticism more suited to an older woman than a flash of too much flesh. Boots have a seductive power in that they guide the eye from the ankle, knee or thigh to hint at, rather than reveal, the pleasures above. As Twiggy says, 'When I see a pair of boots I love, it's very hard for me to walk away' – and there are so many to choose from!

Today Manolo Blahnik, Sergio Rossi, Martine Sitbon and Stephane Kélian are important boot designers; Maurizio Pollini gives the Sixties Chelsea boot a harder, urban edge, while Christian Louboutin makes pairs in violet suede with a rabbit trim and Chloé has boots in white cracked leather. With so many styles to choose from, it's clear that boots are not just items of footwear designed to protect the feet and legs when walking – they are, and have always been, much more.

Glamorous grown-ups wearing boots are refusing to accept the domestic – for who wears boots at home? Boots show intent and what could be more compelling than that? As sixteenth-century philosopher Michel de Montaigne remarked, *'One must always have one's boots on and be ready to go.'* So here's how to get the boots that suit.

BOOTED-UP

THE RIGHT SIZE When comparing shoes to boots, always remember that a shoe has laces or straps to hold the foot in place whereas most boots only have the instep to do the same job. Therefore, a snugger fit is needed. Think about downsizing by about half a size. If your new boots are for winter only and you always wear thick socks with them, don't bother!

THE RIGHT FIT Boots should fit your foot from heel to ball (the widest part). The ball of your foot must match up with the widest part of the outsole and your toes should rest about 2.5 cm (1 in) from the tip of the boot.

THE RIGHT SLIPPAGE You may find that there's a little slippage in the heel of your boot. This doesn't mean that the boot itself doesn't fit – this is completely normal. No slippage probably means the boot is too short and you'll find yourself with a budding blister. As the leather stretches with the form of your foot and the sole begins to flex, slippage will start to disappear. Allow up to two weeks.

THE RIGHT TIGHTNESS The leather of the boot should feel snug across the instep, but not so tight that it pinches. This is vital for a proper fit as the leather will eventually stretch to fit your foot correctly.

★ My calves are so outlandishly fat that it's really difficult to get boots to fit! If your legs are of a similar build, I recommend duoboots.com. Just send in your measurements for a perfect made-to-measure service at a reasonable price to fit any leg. There's a great selection, including glossy black riding boots, biker boots and soft teal suede over-the-knee styles.

★ Decide whether you want a fashion boot or one that works in zero temperatures because they ain't the same thing! Established since 1962, Sorel (sorel.com) produce styles such as the 'Helen of Tundra' and 'Joan of Arctic' for proper snowy winters. More recently, they have attempted to incorporate fashionable features into the boots with rather mixed results.

★ You need spectacular legs to wear an ankle boot with a short skirt. Leave that look to the young and go knee-high instead.

★ Never wear a thigh boot with a short skirt – it's too Julia Roberts in *Pretty Woman* and prospective punters won't look like Richard Gere! In fact, I'm pretty dubious about the whole thigh-high thing on any glamorous grown-up – even Madonna couldn't quite pull off those faux leather Stella McCartney cuissardes. They just look kinda try-hard and icky.

★ Moving on to proportions, take a look at the gap between your skirt and boot – do either of these cut off your leg at the widest part? If you're wearing a longer skirt, make sure the top of it meets the top of your boots. Over-the knee boots that stop just below the hem of the skirt (so no leg at all shows) are very Gucci and perfect for glamorous grown-ups!

★ To elongate your silhouette when booted up, stick to one shade for your skirt, tights (pantyhose) and boots.

───────── ★ ─────────

If you must wear Ugg boots, stick to the real thing and avoid knock-offs – they will lead to what foot experts call the 'Ugg Shuffle', the phrase used to describe the weird lop-sided walk that can ensue when women try to keep the wrong boots on the right feet. The fit is so enormous that your feet slide around so your feet splay and the arches drop, which only exacerbates back problems. We must be careful with wear and tear on our joints as we get older – big, fat Ugg-type boots are so bad for the delicate feet – and also, eventually, the hips – of glamorous grown-ups!

Catherine Zeta-Jones keeps her boots and clothes to a chic black, covers up any hint of bare leg and cleverly streamlines her outfit. Note the eye-wateringly expensive Hermès Kelly.

★ If the zipper won't zip, stop trying – you can't suck in your calves!

★ Avoid patent knee boots but if you're determined to wear them, make sure nothing else shiny is going on with your outfit or you'll look like a stag beetle!

★ Don't wear knee-length boots under jeans – the cuffs may stick out at the knees.

★ Avoid Ugg boots at all costs! They're naff as anything, outsized, outdated, aesthetically tedious and the classic grey 'Cardy' ones simply sear my eyes. They quickly become street-crippled with huge creases at the heels, plus the sides turn over the soles so you find yourself walking on the suede and damaging your feet. Ugg boots are a perfect example of the sartorial distaster that happens when you decide to dress for comfort!

★ Britt Ekland says, 'I know it is incredibly impractical to suggest high heels for walking through the snowy, wintry streets of Stockholm, New York or London. Trying to negotiate snow with ice underneath is lethal, I know. So, go for boots with a wedge heel and non-slip soles. They still give you a bit of a lift.'

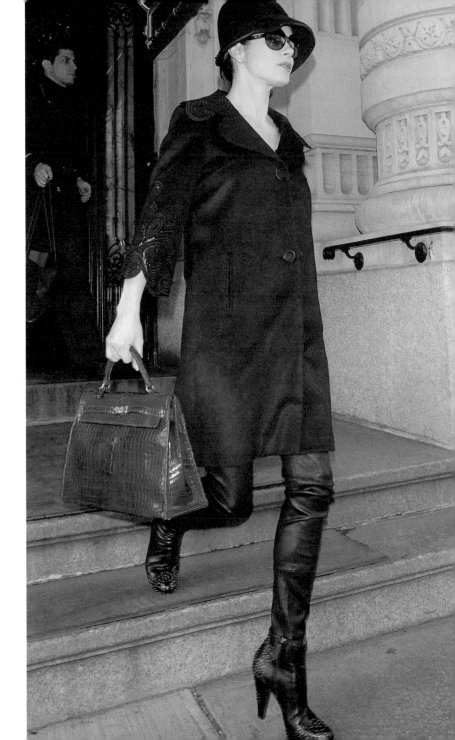

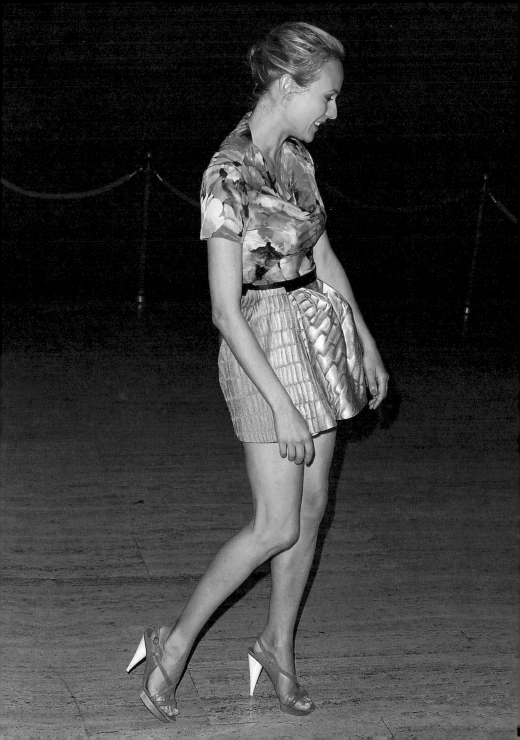

BEST FOOT FORWARD *à la Sophia Loren*

★ 'Avoid white shoes. When a woman wears white shoes they are the only things you see. I watched myself in an early film wearing white pumps and my feet look like Minnie Mouse's – I don't have big feet but those white shoes somehow managed to fill the screen!' (N.B. Heroine Marlene Dietrich agrees, 'White shoes make your feet look large and fat.')

★ 'If you have very nice legs, almost any type of shoe will look pretty on you.'

★ 'Heavy legs or thick ankles are only emphasized by ankle straps – if you have either of these, look for shoes cut low in the front, if possible near the top of the toes. This will give your legs the illusion of length.'

★ 'The best shoe is none at all. Walking in the sand on the beach will suit your feet better than the most expensive shapes – it provides the best possible exercise for feet and legs, firming the muscles while removing rough skin.'

Cross your legs at the ankle instead of the knee when being photographed. It makes your legs look much thinner. Jackie O knew this and when you study any snap of her taken while seated, at least 90 per cent of the time she has her ankles demurely crossed.

This is a clever strappy sandal by Lanvin; the tan tone and platform elongates Diane Kruger's legs whilst the contemporary cone heel is a modern take on an Eighties classic.

3

Let's Get **SKIN DEEP**

We all know that time is a great healer – but it makes a really lousy beautician, and us grown-up girls know that despite our slavish ministrations Nature will always take its course on our visage, no matter how much we try to dodge the thrust of time's arrow. We clearly don't help ourselves with so many midnight assignations in Aspen, fashionable after-parties at the Café de Paris and steamy nights under the stars in St Barts – but when so much is being offered up to us, what's a grown-up girl to do?

On frosty mornings, though, one can feel decidedly *de trop* at the drooping phantom reflected back from the boudoir's Neo-Classical mirror, but that shouldn't mean a frenzied riffling through the back pages of *Vogue* in search of the latest face doc – we are A-List ageless after all and must come to our senses! For in the immortal words of a rooster-cut Rod Stewart, 'The First Cut is the Deepest', and as soon as you've succumbed to the cold steel of the surgeon's knife in that one mad moment of weakness, there really is no going back – just ask Janice Dickinson, whose six-month forays to Dallas for Botox and collagen injections are the stuff of madness.

Pause for thought: time to meditate on taking such a drastic step. Rather than intoning the usual 'Om

Mani Padme Hum' Tibetan mantra, simply chant 'Joan Rivers' for ten minutes. Is her bizarre visage really the one you want to see staring back at you in the bathroom mirror first thing every morning while giving your sparkling pearlies a floss (and that's before we've even got to Priscilla Presley)? It comes to something when even Joan finds her extensive work a little disconcerting, saying, 'I wish I had a twin, then I could know what I'd look like without plastic surgery.' More recently in Hollywood, Joan's whippet in a wind-tunnel facelift has been supplanted by the dreaded 'Pillow Face' or Y-Lift: instead of stretching the skin taut, filler or fat is injected into the cheek area and acts as scaffolding to hold the rest of the face up. The result is, to put it frankly, a bit puffed-up. Stars who are reputed to have had it done recently include Cameron Diaz, Kylie Minogue and Nigella Lawson.

So what's the alternative? To protect and improve the condition of your skin naturally, there are some immediate (and obvious) things you can do that don't involve surgery – as the following pages will attest. Taking care of your skin is not rocket science and involves a series of simple, inexpensive steps that any glamorous grown-up can take.

1 MESSAGE IN A BOTTLE –
Drink Water

Yep, we know it – six to eight glasses a day will keep your skin healthy and glowing. It's kind of weird that a whole designer industry has grown up around something that we can already get out of the tap for free – but that's capitalism for you. If you want to emulate your favourite glamorous grown-up, try these flavours – but remember that in almost every blind tasting test few can distinguish between tap and bottled water.

EVIAN Sooooo Eighties! Raquel Welch reputedly washed her locks in it, Michael Jackson was said to bathe in it and Madonna used to drink it onstage during her Blonde Ambition tour. Who can forget that infamous Evian bottle scene in her 1991 documentary, *Truth or Dare*? Madonna swallows! Also seen in the manicured hands of heroines Michelle Obama and Gwyneth Paltrow.

VOSS Super-premium break through brand from Norway in a distinctive cylindrical glass bottle designed by Neil Kraft, former creative director of Calvin Klein and only available from high-end spas and restaurants. Official bottled water for both the Emmys and Sundance Film Festival and described as 'like drinking fresh air'. If you can be bothered, source a bottle from vossbottledwater.com and then when it's empty, fill straight from the tap!

FIJI You will find bottles of this water in all the rooms and rooftop cabanas at the Peninsula Hotel in Beverly Hills (peninsula.com) and in the designer bags of Jennifer Lopez, Halle Berry and Nicole Kidman. A little pause for thought when you are mid-quaff – although flown straight from Fiji for your delectation, more than half of that island's population has no access to safe and reliable drinking water.

SIGG Your chance to set trends and be eco-friendly at the same time, by filling your personalized bottle with water. This Swiss company dates back to 1908 and their iconic stainless-steel water bottles are a fabulous example of heritage-modern (sigg. com). Recently spotted in the hands of Julia Roberts, Demi Moore, Heidi Klum and Cindy Crawford, the Sigg bottle has a special inner lining that leaves no trace or taint in anything contained inside, won't leach chemicals into water, unlike plastic bottles, and is 100 per cent re-useable as it lasts up to twenty years. What's not to like? (Especially when landfills all over the world are stacked up with plastic water bottles.)

2 *Here Comes the Sun –*
BE A SHADY LADY

The hot rays of the burning sun are always a temptation, but exposure to ultra-violet light is the single thing that ages skin the most. OK, so we're supposed to avoid the sun between 10am and 4pm, sport long sleeves and wide-brimmed hats, and use generous amounts of broad-spectrum suncream, but who cares when you're strapped on the back of a forty-foot floating gin palace reeling in a three-hundred-pound fluorescent marlin off Vanuatu, game fish reel screaming as a muscular deckhand prepares the gaffe? It's the regular prolonged exposure that causes the real problems – a little too much tanning in St Tropez and you could end up like Brigitte Bardot – although she hasn't exactly helped herself by being a smoker, too. Bardot-in-waiting Pamela Anderson is also cracking up a bit and even admits, 'I don't wear sunscreen. I don't have a skin-care programme.'

You should, however, so these are the top five sunscreens.

1 AVÈNE – the best-kept European secret, as used by French madames during their excursions to the Côte d'Azur. The Very High Protection Cream SPF 50 is a 100% mineral sunscreen with a non-irritating, broad spectrum UVA/UVB protection. It's chemical-free and safe for the most sensitive of skins (skinstore.com).

2 LA ROCHE-POSAY ANTHELIOS XL LAIT SPF is recommended by dermatologists because it contains meroxl, a stable sun filter which screens out all those pesky UVA rays that cause wrinkles (laroche-posay.com). Reputedly used by Carla Bruni.

3 VICHY CAPITAL SOLEIL 15 SUNSCREEN CREAM – non-greasy and quickly absorbed into the skin so it doesn't give that heavy, sticky feeling of some other screening products. Ideal for those with easily irritated skin.

4 ELIZABETH ARDEN EIGHT HOUR CREAM SPF 50 SUNSCREEN – broad spectrum with UVA and UVB protection stops skin from becoming dehydrated with humectants such as hyaluronic acid and kinetin, and leaves none of the surfie stoner white residue (shopelizabetharden.com). Used by Victoria Beckham.

5 NEUTROGENA ULTRA SHEER DRY-TOUCH SUNBLOCK – Contains supposedly revolutionary Helioplex technology (what is it with these ad-man names!), a stellar protection against UVA rays. It may be an oil formula but it's not greasy, unlike lots of sunscreens, and it's water resistant so there'll be no eye-stinging when floating off an atoll in the South Pacific (neutrogena.com).

'SUNBURN IS VERY
BECOMING, BUT ONLY
WHEN IT IS EVEN – ONE
MUST BE CAREFUL NOT
TO LOOK LIKE A MIXED GRILL.'

NOEL COWARD

Brigitte Bardot shows how to keep wrinkles at bay – stay in
the shade in a sunhat. Pity she didn't keep this habit up, as
her St Tropez tanning habit has caused visible skin damage.

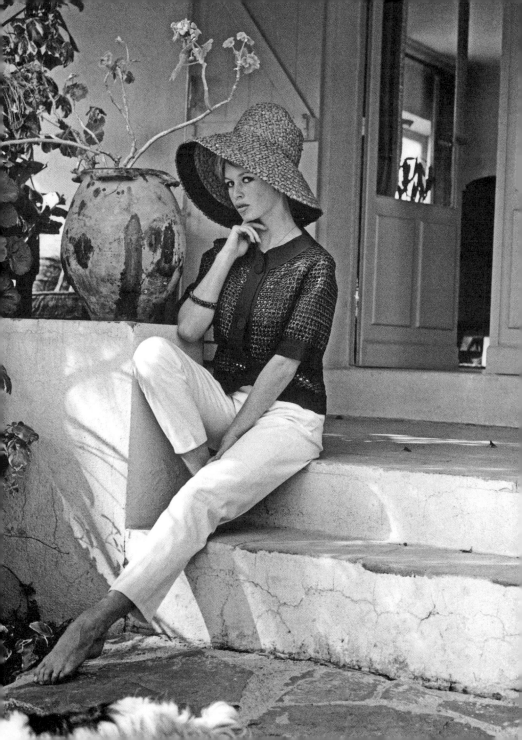

3 *It's a Drag (but)* – **STOP SMOKING**

C'mon people, why bother drinking litres of Pure Samoa Water if you're still chuffing away on the cheroots? I know that for some, a cigarette is a portable therapist but those little suckers wreak havoc on your skin by speeding up the ageing process. Face facts: the more gaspers you smoke, and the longer you keep up the habit, the more wrinkles you will have – not just on your face but on your neck, hands and inner arms, too.

Nicotine causes the blood vessels in the outermost layers of your skin to narrow. The result is de-oxygenated and nutrient-starved skin. Chemicals contained in tobacco smoke also harm collagen and elastin, the fibres that give your skin its strength and elasticity – ironically, the self-same ones that you are trying to repair with expensive anti-ageing unguents.

Warning! Pursing your lips while inhaling and squinting your eyes to prevent the sting of tobacco smoke may look good on Clint Eastwood in *The Outlaw Josey Wales*, but it's less impressive on a sophisticated femme fatale.

Nicotine addiction can also be a bit tricky – once, when on an American Airlines flight, Whitney Houston crept off to the plane's powder room because she was desperate to spark up a ciggie – ooh the glamour! The captain was called and soberly informed her that if she went ahead, it would cost her a cool $2,000 in fines. Whitney, ever the diva, went to write the cheque, but the captain refused to back down.

A Daily DOSE

Skin supplements in pill form help from the inside out while also improving your general wellbeing, especially those that contain essential omega-3 fat supplement, vitamin C and minerals.

TOP THREE SUPPLEMENTARY BENEFITS

1 IMEDEEN, actually an extract of fish cartilage, is said to help with reducing fine lines (although according to the British Dermatological Foundation there has been only one study to suggest this and it was carried out on just 30 women). Imedeen can be taken in supplement form alongside your usual skincare regime. (Imedeen Time Perfection for 40+ imodeen.co.uk)

2 DR MURAD YOUTH BUILDER contains glucosamine and amino acids designed to boost collagen and increase the skin's elasticity. (murad.com)

3 BEAUTY SCOOP is a drinkable powder that purports to contain all you need for great skin and hair. There's a big buzz about it at the moment but it's not cheap! (beautyscoop.com)

TOP TIP

PERFECTIL PLUS is a personal favourite – not least because it's cheap! Contains fatty acids, which boost hydration and help with UV damage. (vitabiotics.com)

HOPE *in a Jar*

Beauty's holy grail: a little pot of unction to turn back time and for the manufacturers, a billion-dollar business.

It's a bamboozling minefield out there – serums, extracts, enhancers and boosters all described in quasi-scientific language by hatchet-faced beauty assistants in white lab coats, who try to convince us that this stuff actually works. But have you really noticed what they look like? Is there a global directive that insists women on the luxury brand counters in Harvey Nicks/Barneys/Printemps must trowel on all the make-up ranges at once? It's a no-win situation for us grown-up girls – we have to decide whether we are prepared to part with squillions for a pot of Crème de Mer, a financial investment in our facial future, but we can't claim our cash back if it doesn't work. Maybe the psychology of buying a pot of expensive cream is the same as investing in a fabulous perfume – it may not have any effect other than psychological and, ye gods, there's nothing wrong with that in our troubled times! But I'd rather spend it on a weekend away looking at Gaudí and sharing tapas with a sweaty gaucho in Barcelona.

Do any magic line blitzers really work? Very few have been scientifically tested, with the exception of Boots No7 Protect & Perfect Beauty Serum. Stocks sold out after Professor Chris Griffiths, Foundation Professor of Dermatology at Manchester University said: 'At both basic science and clinical levels Boots No7 Protect & Perfect has been shown scientifically to repair photo-aged skin and improve the fine wrinkles associated with photo-ageing.' This statement followed the first proper trial of an over-the-counter cosmetics product as opposed to drugs such as Tretinoin, which are only available on prescription.

It may be a bitter pill for some of us to swallow but there is no long-lasting, conclusive way to prevent wrinkles developing without the intervention of major surgery – but that, of course, makes you look mad. It's time to move on! If you have nothing better to do than obsessively scan in the mirror for signs of decay (c'mon people!), look for skin creams or gels containing Vitamin A or retinol – this is the magic ingredient and it comes in a variety of mild forms – retinoids – which seem to have an effect on fine lines. Stronger retinol can only be obtained on prescription and includes tazarotene gel and tretinoin, aka Retin-A, which works by stimulating your skin to produce collagen and helps new skin cells to grow while replacing older ones. It can have side effects such as irritation, though, and you will need to avoid the sun. Many over-the-counter crèmes now contain retinol, some with more than others.

————★————

BOOTS NO7 PROTECT & PERFECT INTENSE BEAUTY SERUM is a more intense version for grown-up skins and contains a greater number of the line-busting ingredients.

The best include:

★ **SKINCEUTICALS RETINOL 0.5** (skinceuticals.com)

★ **LA ROCHE-POSAY BIOMEDIC RETINOL 15** (laroche-posay.com)

★ **AFIRM 3X** (dermstore.com)

Heroine SKINCARE TIPS

★ **MARILYN MONROE** used a satin pillowcase to prevent wrinkles. Silk absorbs less moisture than cotton and helps keep your skin hydrated when you sleep. The friction created by cotton leaves more creases in your skin! Silk also prevents bed-head.

★ **JENNIFER ANISTON** says it's all about soap: 'I wash with the same soap that I have since I was a teenager, which is Neutrogena. And that's it!'

★ **PENELOPE CRUZ** says the secret to flawless skin is sleep. *'Sleep is the best way to happiness and beauty. Once, my sister slept for three days straight. My record is 18 hours, though I don't usually sleep that long.'*

★ **HALLE BERRY** recommends having a baby when in your forties (?!): 'I have so much joy and energy. I can just go and go and go, my skin is aglow from all the hormones. I actually wear less make-up now, which is really good.'

★ **NIGELLA LAWSON**: *'I think what ages a face most is disappointment and a lack of enjoyment so I try to do what I love.'*

Penelope Cruz's tip for beautiful skin is simple – a good night's sleep. And as a spokeswoman for L'Oreal she must get loads of free products!

★ Advice according to **TERI HATCHER**: 'When you're alone, open a bottle of wine. This make-up chemist that I know was talking about all the good properties in wine – antioxidants and stuff, exfoliating qualities – and she said: "Never throw it out, dump it in your bath." It makes you feel luxurious.'

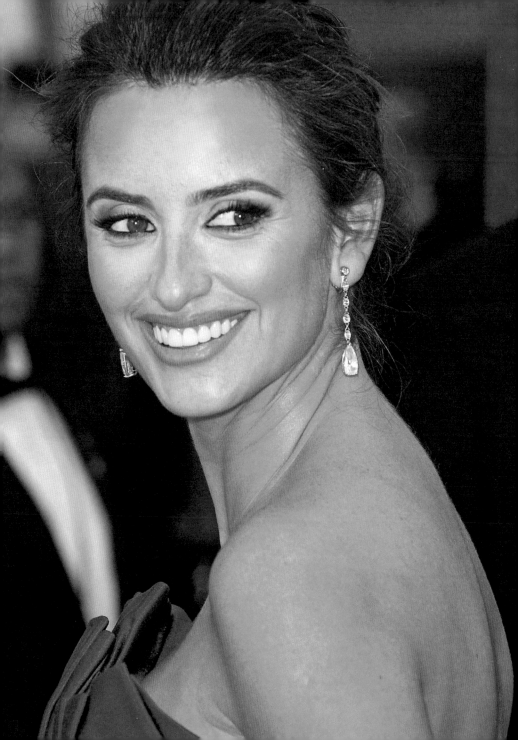

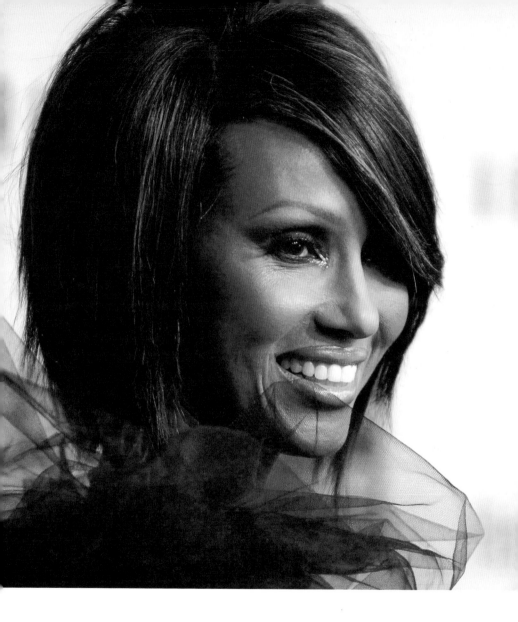

★ **CLAUDIA SCHIFFER** says, 'I still believe that drinking at least a litre of water and several cups of peppermint tea a day is the easiest way to make your skin glow.'

★ **ESTEE LAUDER** always advised never to leave the house without wearing a hat – '*You only get one face. Protect it.*'

★ **IMAN**'s secret? '*Skincare, skincare, skincare! Look after your skin in your teens and 20s because it's the one you inherit in your 50s and beyond.*'

★ **SHARON STONE**: 'My mother gave me a jar of Avon Rich Moisture Cream when I was 14. She said, "Don't ask me why – but you'll thank me later."'

★ It's all about mood according to **CATE BLANCHETT**: 'My skin improves when I'm happy.'

★ Finally, **COCO CHANEL**: '*Nature gives you the face you have at twenty. Life shapes the face you have at thirty. But at fifty you get the face you deserve.*'

Iman says that for an older woman 'skincare comes first' and 'use an SPF under your foundation, despite how dark you are. The sun does not discriminate, ladies!'

HOW TO GET *an A-List Facial*

A week before Oscar night, Susan Sarandon, Rachel Weisz, Meryl Streep and Kate Winslet all book into Tracie Martyn's 59 Fifth Avenue Spa, New York for a Resculpting Facial.

Like a gym for the face, Martyn's facial is a magical mix of micro dermabrasion, mild electric currents and a hydrating aromatic oxygen bath. It's a compelling combination of green-ness (the products are organic and include fruit enzymes, plant extracts and peptides) and new technology. Grown-up girls swear by it – Kate Winslet insists: 'It makes you look brighter, healthier … like you got some extra rest.' Diane von Furstenberg and Susan Sarandon have been advocates for ten years.

British-born Martyn, aka Facialist to the Stars, was originally a make-up artist who began giving pre-shoot facials in her Brookyn-based apartment. Her pre-event treatments for stars such as Penelope Cruz were so successful she branched out into organic skincare combined with mild electric treatment and dermabrasion to polish the skin, dubbed by John Galliano, 'the haute couture of treatments'. There's also a Martyn outpost at Lapis The Spa at the Fontainebleu Hotel.

Martyn products are widely available (traceymartyn.com). The Anti-ageing Amla purifying cleanser is good for cleansing and exfoliating without stripping the skin. It's a tad expensive but you only use a small amount and its citrus smell is lovely.

HOW TO DO *a DIY Facial*

You can give yourself a purifying steam facial at home that will help not only your skin but also your stress levels.

Wear a head-band to keep your hair away from your face. Remove all traces of make-up so your skin is squeaky clean.

Fill a large bowl with hot water, heated enough so that the steam will last for about five minutes, to which you have added a couple of pinches of loose green tea, then hold your face over the steam about a foot from the bowl whilst covering your head with a towel. Stop if it feels too hot and wait for the water to cool down a bit!

─────★─────

The first time you have a steam facial you will get a few blemishes; this is natural and the more you do it the more your skin will improve. Steam your face in moderation if you have dry or sensitive skin.

You can alternatively add mint, rosemary or lavender oil – or even a chamomile teabag, but make sure you steep it in a cup first and then add the water to the bowl.

Pat your face dry with a clean towel and then apply a very light moisturiser to your face.

THE 'IT' *Face*

★ **CLARA BOW** – Chipmunk cheeks matched with full pouting lower lip.

★ **GRACE KELLY** – Waspy patrician with the perfect ski-jump nose.

★ **AUDREY HEPBURN** – Bambi eyes set almost halfway down her strangely compressed face.

★ **BRIGITTE BARDOT** – Lavish lips and a cute button nose, the perfect sex kitten.

★ **TWIGGY** – An oval face, wide-set eyes and pouting lower lip, more Renaissance than sixties.

★ **CHERYL TIEGS** – High cheekbones and square jaw heralded American athleticism.

★ **CHRISTY TURLINGTON** – Spookily symmetrical, this beautiful alien has an oval face perfectly divided up into thirds – forehead/eyes and cheekbones/ generous mouth.

★ **ANGELINA JOLIE** – Unusually deep-set eyes mixed with razor-sharp cheekbones, extraordinary lips and a strong jawline.

Christy Turlington, the model whose perfectly balanced face defined the Eighties, says, 'My face is a dime a dozen in many parts of the world.' After modelling she studied for a masters degree in public health at Columbia University.

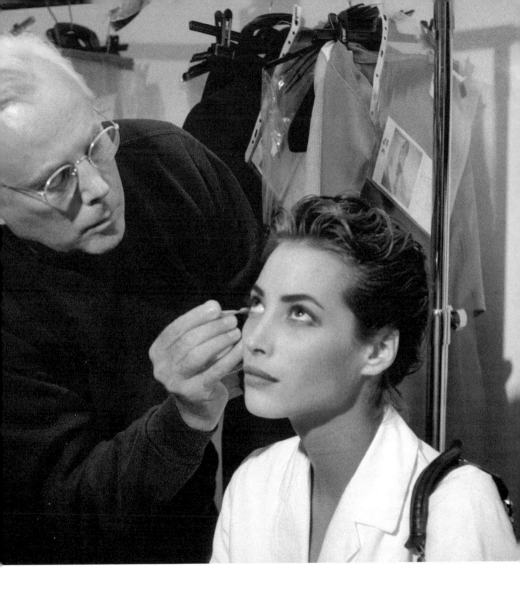

HOW I LEARNED *To Love My Neck*

Jeez, what's happening to my neck? It's kinda gone all wobbly in the middle and my face and neck are fast becoming one, fusing together in a bizarre tube of flesh! Why did no one tell me this would happen? Necks have thinner skin than the face and less fat and oil glands, which is why they tend to go first. As heroine Nora Ephron says, 'Our faces are lies and our necks are the truth. You have to cut open a redwood tree to see how old it is, but you wouldn't if it had a neck.'

I have come to realize that there is nothing much I can do about it, but my decaying neck is the perfect excuse for another vintage Hermès scarf or Robert Larin pendant. If thy neck offends thee, maybe these tips could help:

★ Don't stop at the jawline – keep moisturizing downwards, but apply with upward strokes! If you are pernickety about the right product for the right bit, then buy special neck creams that target this area – but by the time you've done your face, then under-eye, the serum, the blah, you will have lost all will (and several hours of blissful sleep). Many recommend the Pevonia Botanica Restore Neck & Bust Cream (pevonia. com), 3Lab Perfect Neck Cream (3lab.com) and Decleor Excellence de L'Age Neck Cream (decleor.co.uk).

★ Wear sunscreen every day, all year round – the neck has some of the most delicate tissues on it so if you're slathering your face, do the same to your neck.

★ Stop smoking or you'll get a crepey, creepy lizard neck.

★ Posture makes a world of a difference – hold your head up!

★ Before investing too much money on any beauty product, study the on-line reviews first. There are so many beauty blogs out there, such as beautyandthedirt.com, ciao.co.uk and make-upalley.com. You can easily find the right product for your skin type – and get the lowdown on whether brands are exaggerating the claims they make for their products!

★ Facial exercises will firm the jowels, so close your lips and pull up the corners of your mouth into a wide smile. Inhale through your nose and, at the same time, look up, thereby stretching your neck and throat. Hold this pose for as long as possible, then slowly exhale as you release and relax your face and neck muscles. Repeat this foolishness at least ten times.

★ The muscle in the neck is called the platysma and when it weakens with age it separates in the middle to give the dreaded turkey wattle effect. To firm up this area tilt your head as far back as possible and press your tongue into the roof of your mouth. Bring your chin down whilst holding your tongue in place. If there is a feeling of tightness under your chin and at the front of your neck you are doing the exercise correctly.

★ A polo neck is an obvious choice for neck disguise but it does not suit the large busted and if there is any flesh on your chin it will be pushed upwards, causing instant fatness. A cowl neck is a much better option and a less obvious 'I'm disguising my neck' disguise.

IN YOUR FACE! *The Perils of Botox*

A botulism-based wrinkle eradicator has swept the world, causing grown women to eat organic food while having poison injected into their face. So, what's going on? All you need to know is that large quantities of Botox over several years atrophy the facial muscles, so you end up looking like a partially defrosted cryogenic experiment. The benefits of Botox are only temporary, so you've wasted your money and now you're walking round with an immobile flat forehead that looks permanently saturated in oil because of the way light bounces off it! The area across the top of your nose has widened so strangely that you look like a fish.

Susan Sarandon says that she has 'nothing against people doing it, but I need my face to move. I was watching a movie, and I couldn't figure out what was so odd. Then I realized the poor actress was howling, but nothing was moving. It gives a very Kabuki-esque edge to the performance.'

If that hasn't put you off, visit realself.com/Botox/reviews where punters will give you the lowdown on their latest jabs.

Susan Penhaligon, hailed in the seventies as the British answer to Bardot, had Botox at the age of 60: 'I was a complete wally to have it in the first place. It very nearly had a disastrous effect on my career and on my confidence as a person. I will never go near it again.'

Glamorous Grown-Ups **TALK SURGERY**

SUSAN SARANDON: 'I don't like it when surgeons take a perfectly interesting-looking woman and she ends up looking like a female impersonator with these gigantic breasts. It's just so extreme and that worries me.'

ROSANNA ARQUETTE: 'Look, it's got to the point where kids are getting Botox. It's insane. We're not allowed to age.'

KATE WINSLET: *'I'd like to grow old with my face moving.'*

CATHERINE DENEUVE: 'Actresses have to be able to frown.'

CATE BLANCHETT: I see someone's face, someone's body who has had children, and I think they're the song lines of your experience, and why would you want to eradicate that?'

HALLE BERRY: 'I hope I will evolve as a person who realizes it's really not about my physical appearance and not be drawn to that seductive knife.'

JENNIFER ANISTON: *'I tried Botox once. I felt like I had a weight on my head.'*

TERI HATCHER: 'I don't use Botox or Restylane and I've never had any surgery, no matter what you've read.'

REGRETS? *I've Had a Few...*

'If anyone says their facelift doesn't hurt, they're lying. It was like I'd spent the night with an axe murderer.'
SHARON OSBOURNE

'I've been on the cover of every magazine in the world but as a young model, I never felt as beautiful as I looked. I masked it well with alcoholism. I grew up in an abusive home and was told on a daily basis by my father that I would never amount to anything and that I looked like a boy. One of the main reasons I had a lot of plastic surgery was because of the voice of my father. I've had my boobs and eyes done, my forehead lifted, and my stomach done. I'm addicted to cosmetic surgery! But plastic surgery hasn't stifled the voice from my father.'
JANICE DICKINSON

'The trouble with plastic surgery is that after ten years, gravity wins out and you have to have another one in a year or so.'
LINDA EVANS

'We've got into this state where women see a problem and their first thought is surgery. It's so wrong. I look for alternatives. Recently I was at a spa and had a frozen-water treatment that firmed everything up. Amazing! I took a packet of frozen peas and placed them under my eyes for a few minutes. It works. Acupuncture facials work. Body-brushing works. Exercise works. Not drinking and not smoking works. Facials work, for God's sake.'
SADIE FROST

‘COSMETIC SURGERY IS TERRIFYING. IT NEVER LOOKS GOOD. THOSE WOMEN LOOK WEIRD. THEY LOOK IN THE MIRROR AND THINK THEY LOOK GREAT, BUT THEY DON'T SEE WHAT WE SEE. IT'S HIDEOUS. THEY SCARE SMALL CHILDREN.’

JERRY HALL

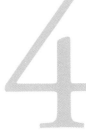

LESS IS MORE
The New Rules of Make-up

As the great French couturier Yves Saint Laurent once said, 'The most beautiful make-up of a woman is passion. But cosmetics are easier to buy.' Well, all I can add is, thank God for maquillage! It can perk up the most crumbling of visages and gives hope to the hungover. As Bette Davis drawled, 'I will not retire while I've still got my legs and my make-up box.'

As we change, so too should our make-up, but some grown-up girls get stuck in the same old routine with Seventies snail-trail highlighters and cherry-flavoured gloss – more Coco the Clown than Coco Chanel. Yet A-List make-up gives any face an instant 'lift' – you just have to know what works for you. The problem is being surrounded by such a vast array of available products in the stores. It can be more than a tad daunting, even for Sandra Bullock who confesses, 'Make-up is scary. When I do it myself, it's just mascara, and sometimes I forget even to do that.' What hope have we when she has beauty professionals at her beck and call?

So, let's get down to basics. For glamorous grown-ups the key message is 'Less is More' – too much make-up looks too tranny. For ageless glamour, understatement is the golden rule. 'The best thing is to look natural,' says Calvin Klein, 'but it takes make-up to look natural.' And as supermodel Lauren Hutton points out, 'The mistake women make is you shouldn't see your make-up. We don't want to look like we've made an effort.' What must be borne in mind is that what constitutes a natural look differs from era to era, evidence the films set in the past that always reflect the era in which they were made – think actress Faye Dunaway embodying late Sixties cool in *Bonnie and Clyde*, set in 1930s Depression-hit Oklahoma.

OK, so a 'natural' look provided by cosmetics is something of an oxymoron, but a natural effect can be achieved by a barely-there, subtle application of the best that the cosmetic chemist has to offer. It's to do with concealing and enhancing, not exaggerating.

EYES *Right!*

Helena Rubenstein once said, '*Adjust your make-up to the light in which you wear it*' and I can second that while emphasizing that you must never use any product with twinkly-dinkly sparkles in it. Any degree of shimmer will cling to your creases, like Paris Hilton to a goodie bag.

Avoid multi-tonal palettes; you'll be tempted to use the irridescent shades that come in them and one day, in a moment of weakness, you'll pick it up and go, 'Ooh, that looks nice!' – it doesn't. Always buy single shades – MAC do the best (maccosmetics.com for stockists). While you're at it, ditch the pale blue eye shadow! Brown can be beyond dreary every day and can even make you look a little downbeat. As eyes get older, they tend to become more deep-set and therefore look smaller. Perk 'em up with one of Bobbi Brown's duo-sets of subtle colours that are perfect for grown-up glamour without being too obtrusive. Order on-line at bobbibrown.co.uk.

Kate Winslet in her favourite make-up combo: peach eye-shadow and blush, fine liquid eyeliner, not too much mascara and well defined brows. Her lips are almost always neutral or slightly darker than her natural colour.

All eye shadow needs to be applied over a primer, which forms the perfect base for colour. Primer is a modern product that actually works far better than the old method of using foundation or concealer and does a double job of eradicating dark shadows and ensures that the eye shadow goes on evenly. By far the best (honestly, I haven't got shares in the company) is Bobbi Brown's Tinted Eye Brightener cream, which now comes in a portable stick form. Personally, I prefer using the old brush method – it's a more versatile method of application and can really get into the eye socket.

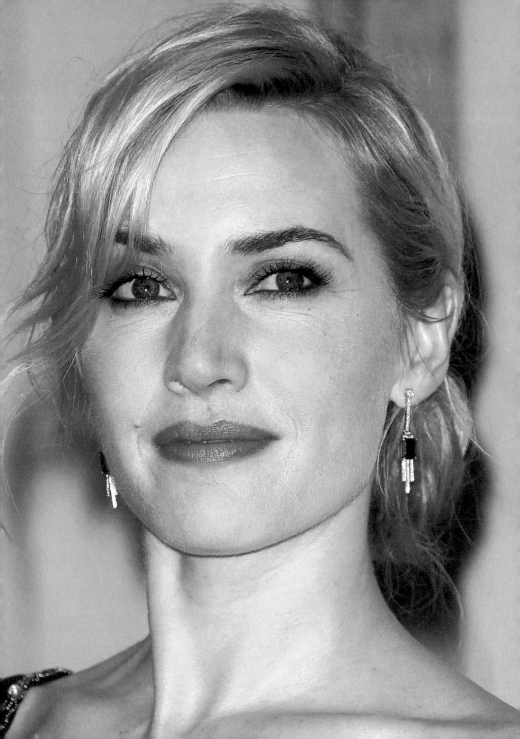

International make-up artist Daniel Kolaric says: 'The skin under your eyes is much finer than on the rest of your face so you will need to start using eye cream as you get older. Standard moisturizer remains greasy under your eyes because the skin cannot absorb it, the result is eye make-up sliding down your face.'

———————— ★ ————————
Once you have applied eye shadow, add a little eye brightener to the outside edge of the eye for an instant lift to those droopy corners.

Mascara needs to make your eyelashes look like an intense version of the natural you. Use black, brown and dark navy only – no silly colours allowed – and avoid clumpiness by brushing out the excess with a clean baby toothbrush. Mascara recipes and techniques for applying it are changing all the time and include vibrating wands and sputnik-shaped brushes to reach the tiny lashes in the inner corner of the eyes. L'Oréal are renowned for mascara innovation: a recent double-ended version offers a renewal lash serum to nourish your lashes, which is intended to be worn underneath mascara. The serum is at one end and the ultra-lengthening mascara at the other. If you can't be bothered with all that, stick with tried and true staples such as Maybelline Great Lash with its distinctive pink and green bottle, as worn by Linda Evangelista and Christy Turlington – easy, effective and waterproof.

Always use eyelash curlers on clean lashes, an instrument that looks as if it belongs in a medieval torture chamber but really opens up the eyes.

'I DON'T BELIEVE MAKE-UP
AND THE RIGHT HAIRSTYLE
ALONE CAN MAKE A
WOMAN BEAUTIFUL. THE
MOST RADIANT WOMAN
IN THE ROOM IS THE ONE
FULL OF LIFE AND EXPERIENCE.'

SHARON STONE

TOP THREE *Wrinkle Primer Gels*

★ **DIOR'S MULTI-PERFECTION RADIANCE ENHANCER** does what it says on the tin: smooths, evens and brightens. Expensive, but worth it!

★ **SEPHORA IMMEDIATE WRINKLE FILLER** (sephora.com) gets genuinely good reviews and is great round the lips to prevent lipstick feathering. Make sure you blend the gel in really well, though, or it can leave strange white flaky patches!

★ **CLARINS INSTANT SMOOTH PERFECTING TOUCH** (available at most department stores or online) is fantastic on most skin types. Make sure you wait a minute so that it's absorbed into the skin before applying foundation.

For spectacular, yet natural results, try eyelash extensions. Initially treated as a joke and one step too far in the high maintenance stakes, eyelash extensions are, in fact, so effective that you can ditch all other eye make-up for a completely natural look. Unlike false lashes with their cheesy connotations of Sixties' dolly birds and today's D-List boilers, extensions make the eyes look alert, sparkling and youthful. Each fake lash is individually bonded to your own and the effect lasts for four to six weeks provided you do not use an oil-based make-up remover. Applying a full set of 80 eyelashes takes just under an hour and is a service available in most local beauty salons.

——————★——————

Most women need reading glasses to correct the long-sightedness that comes with growing up. Such lenses enlarge the look of the eye, and therefore exaggerate the amount and effect

Don't use eyeliner under your eyes at all – it will make any eye look smaller.

of eye make-up. Frames can make a huge difference to the youthful appearance of the face, providing instant dowdiness or, conversely, extreme hotness. They are an accessory, and therefore need to be updated, so keep an eye on current trends. Don't be tempted to use glasses that disappear – colourless frames and grey hair will render you invisible. Never, never, never wear them on a chain around your neck – ever! And try not to peer over the top of them.

A HINT *of Tint*

In the summer, when my skin tones even out,
I prefer to use a sheer tinted moisturizer plus
concealer instead of foundation. You need one
that will cover yet also hydrate your skin without
looking greasy. Lancôme Aqua Fusion Teinté SPF
15 is one of the best out there (lancome.co.uk).
Bobbi Brown also provides a SPF of 25 in her
luxuriously textured Tinted Moisturizing Balm –
perfect for summer sun.

Occasionally, I also use a wrinkle primer gel under
the tinted moisturizer as it seems to smooth out
the skin and lasts all day. Daniel Kolaric says,
'Many primer gels have light-reflecting particles
that bounce light off the skin. Discoloration and
an uneven skin surface appear more ageing than
mere wrinkles, hence the preoccupation by beauty
companies to even out colour and emphasize
texture instead.'

A Firm **FOUNDATION**

Don't be afraid to use foundation. If your memories of foundation are orange streaks along the jawline, pores as open as Jack Nicholson's Y-fronts and a ghastly chalkiness to the cheeks, take another look. New generation foundations are superb. The older skin of us grown-up girls needs coverage; age spots and broken capillaries, particularly around the nose, can't be obscured by a little tinted moisturizer and a dab of powder. Modern foundations are not just skin enhancers: they provide all-important protection from the sun and should ideally be applied over moisturizer and a skin serum. Do not aim for a flat, matt surface coverage, these products give a fresh, dewy youthful luminescence that has to be seen to be believed!

1 All foundation samples that come attached to magazine advertisements are usually far too dark.

2 Seek professional advice in a department store for your shade if you're a novice at this make-up lark!

3 Never use foundation beneath your eyes – it will make the delicate skin look like crepe paper.

Dior make the Rolls-Royce of foundations – the magnificent Capture Totale can be found in most department stores or online. The downside is that it's madly expensive (you could make a case for it by telling yourself that it contains a skin serum so you have two products in one and you don't have to use that much). Chanel Mat Lumière fluid make-up is an excellent alternative for grown-up skin, although it has a tendency to cause breakouts if your complexion is oily. Follow this with a mineral face powder applied with a brush and the all-important blusher.

BLUSH *or Flush?*

Use blusher! As we ripen, we lose pigment from our skin and can look pale and washed-out rather than pale and interesting if we don't add a bit of colour to our cheeks. Blusher will make you appear much fresher, but don't overdo it – you don't want to be rushed to a burns unit!

Never underestimate the power of pink on the older skin and avoid anything remotely tawny, or you'll look like you haven't washed your face properly. Powder blushes are good, but seem to linger as long as Britney's latest beau and need constant reapplying. I find that stains, gels and liquid blushers dry quickly and become extremely hard to manipulate (like my latest beau), so the new combination powder creams are better for that much-needed 'pop' of colour. A favourite to replicate one's youthful rosy glow is Nars Blush in Orgasm (narscosmetics.com).

THE NEW RULES OF BLUSHER

1 Apply all blusher to the apples of your cheeks (the place that swells when you smile).

2 If you are going through the hot flush phase, don't be tempted to eschew blusher. Each sweaty rush is momentary, so ride it out and the blush on your cheek will keep you looking cool.

3 For the perfect finish, apply a very small amount of MAC's Strobe Cream over your blusher. Rub it into the palm of one hand and pat the cheeks gently for a light-enhancing finish.

Sarah Jessica Parker's
TOP FIVE BEAUTY PRODUCTS

1 C.O. BIGELOW ROSE SALVE
(bigelowchemists.com): 'I apply it to my
lips every night before bed. It has the most
amazing smell.'

2 SHISEIDO PURENESS CLEANSING FOAM
(ciao.co.uk): 'I always think things get cleaner if the
formula gets foamy. I'm sure that's not scientifically
true, but I love the bubbles!'

3 KERASTASE MASQUE OLEO-RELAX
(luxuryhaircare.co.uk): 'This is not cheap stuff, but
it really does terrific things for my hair.'

4 BUMBLE AND BUMBLE SUNDAY SHAMPOO
(hair-care.co.uk): 'It gives my hair that squeaky
clean feeling that I've loved ever since I was a child.'

5 GARNIER NUTRITIONISTE ULTRA-LIFT PRO CREAM
(garnier.com): 'This targets all the things that are
important to treat someone my age, like dryness
and wrinkles.'

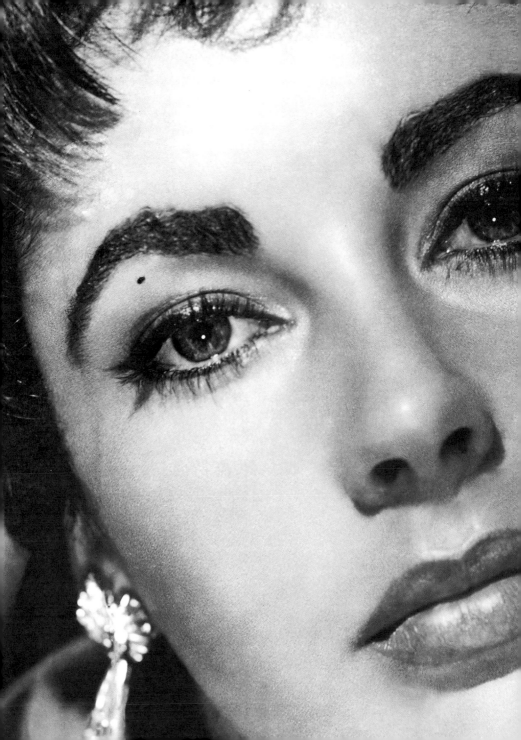

HIGH BROW *Eyebrows*

A good eyebrow shape is essential whether you prefer to look natural or not because it can really define the face and lift the eyes, if treated with right respect. Fashions in brows come and go, moving from thick to thin and back again during the decades. If you haven't changed your shape for years, take heed: get plucked, and if you're still a bushy Brooke Shields, and if you think thin is in, then you're waaaay out.

Time is not kind to our brows. They tend to thin to the point of invisibility, or become as unruly and grey as a badger's. It is tempting to pluck out the odd grey hair but you must resist – you will only be left with a bald patch. Get out an eyebrow kit and tint 'em instead! And for the love of God, don't tattoo eyebrows on. You might be thinking Catherine Zeta-Jones, but it'll turn out Michael Jackson. As our faces begin to follow the laws of gravity, your eyebrows will stay where they are and the most permanent thing on your face will be a startled expression. BTW: black tattooed brows fade to a light biro blue!

———— ★ ————

Plucking never hurts as much if someone does it for you. When you do it yourself, you anticipate the pain! It's always better to pluck after showering because your skin is softer and more malleable then.

BTW It's also a myth that you should never pluck hairs from the top of your eyebrows – as you get older, you'll find that more grow there and for a perfect arch, they need to go! Slant tweezers are the most effective and Tweezerman do the best. (tweezerman.com)

Elizabeth Taylor's eyebrows were a perfect match for her oval face and intense violet eyes. In 1976 she won the title of Most Memorable Eyebrows in a magazine poll – the first runner up was Lassie!

HERE'S HOW TO GET THE PERFECT EYEBROWS:

STEP 1 Stand in a good light – daylight is by far the best – and use a decently sized magnifying mirror rather than squinting like Blind Pugh through your compact.

STEP 2 With white eyebrow pencil in hand, begin on the right: place it vertically along the side of your nose so that it juts up just past your brow. Any stray hairs between the pencil and the bridge of your nose must go, but remember to always pluck the hair in the direction that it grows.

STEP 3 Now place the pencil diagonally so it rests at the edge of your nostril to meet the outer corner of your eye. Little pesky hairs below the pencil should be taken out, too.

STEP 4 Now here comes the tricky bit! Look steadily right into the mirror and place the pencil vertically along the outer part of your iris. Take out any stray hairs lying beneath the natural arch. This will have the most amazing effect of opening up your eyes. Just compare with the un-plucked one and you will see the miraculous result! Repeat with the other eyebrow.

STEP 5 Add definition with an eyebrow brush and pencil. Take the brush and brush your eyebrows downwards and then add colour (a warm brown or taupe suits most people) carefully along the top of your brows. Brush your eyebrows back and then fill in underneath with feathery strokes – your brows should look more naturally defined.

STEP 6 Hold the colour fast with brow gel.

PLAN YOUR OWN SALON
by Mala Rubinstein

Decide on the area where your beauty rituals will take place and equip it as efficiently and as prettily as a small salon. Whether it is your bathroom, dressing room or bedroom, store your beauty essentials in an easily accessible place. Line up jars and bottles in the order in which you use them. Keep all containers neat, smudge-free and appealing!

Have tissues and cotton wool close at hand. Include among the essentials a headband to tie back and protect your hair whenever you are caring for your skin or applying make-up, plus a plastic cape or make-up bib. When the atmosphere of your 'beauty salon' is as pretty and feminine as you yourself, your daily programme will be more enjoyable – and perhaps even more fruitful.'

A Little LIP ACTION

As we grow older, even the most Jolie-esque of lips begin to thin and lose their pout, usually as a result of sun damage (yeah, that again!) and the gradual slowing down of the production of collagen and elastin. Colour tends to fade, too, and as little wrinkles appear on the lip line, the contour of your mouth tends to lack a little definition. All is not lost, though, as there are actually many things you can do to get your lips back in good smooching order that don't involve the pout de trout.

Injectible lip fillers such as Restylane may be fashionable but I have never, ever seen them used successfully and there is nothing worse than seeing a once-gorgeous woman inflate her lips to porn-star proportions. Meg Ryan looks like she has a pair of greasy hot dogs attached to her face and there is something peculiar about seeing Nicole Kidman's lips appear to turn inside out when she smiles. Viewed from the side, their mouths are even more of a mess and the lumpy unevenness of some stars' pouts makes them look as if they've done battle with fish bait or are using Marge Simpson as a role model. There are other options to give yourself fuller, more natural-looking lips that might not have such instant gratification but at least fishermen won't attempt to harpoon you!

★

Ashley Judd rubs a couple of pineapple chunks over her lips to slough off the dead skin, then follows up with a dab of petroleum jelly to seal in the moisture.

PUCKER *Up*

You probably already exfoliate your face, but don't forget your lips, too. Regular exfoliation will remove dead skin cells and gives you a truly kissable pout. Your lips will also be less prone to chapping and hold lipstick for longer.

STEP 1 Buy a soft-bristled toothbrush and designate this only for your lips.

STEP 2 Apply a warm damp flannel to your lips for a couple of minutes.

STEP 3 Run your toothbrush under a lukewarm tap then shake off the excess moisture.

STEP 4 Apply an exfoliant. There are a myriad of products you can use – a light application of toothpaste, a sugar and honey mix (which you can eat afterwards, yum!) or simply Vaseline will all lightly buff your lips.

STEP 5 Use the toothbrush to massage your lips softly in small, circular motions for a minute.

STEP 6 Gently rinse and then apply lip balm or Vaseline.

TOP FIVE *Lip Exfoliants*

If you are crazy for products and find my cheap and cheerful alternatives lack the appropriate glamour for your Philippe Starck wet room, try the following:

1 LAURA MERCIER LIP SILK

(lauramercier.com). Exfoliates and moisturizes to leave lips as soft as silk. Stops lipstick feathering around the mouth.

2 PETER THOMAS ROTH LIPS TO DIE FOR

(peterthomasroth.com) Genius three-step system made up of a sugary lemony exfoliating scrub, followed by a Lip Putty (basically a mud mask that you rinse off with warm water) and finally, the Pink Bombshell Lip Balm. Definitely perked up my pout!

3 LEAF AND RUSHER TX LIPS

(leafandrusher.com) Anti-ageing lip product from Beverly Hills – exfoliates and plumps with a pleasant sugary aftertaste.

4 SMASHBOX EMULSION LIP EXFOLIANT

(smashbox.com) Cooling sugar and peppermint scrub with shea butter.

PLUMP *Up*

Lip plumpers are an easy and safe, if short-term solution for lips that need a little pre-party help, but they are not something that I would use every day. Many have ingredients which purport to help stimulate collagen production, but approach these with a degree of scepticism. What makes a plumper work in the short term is the mild stimulant they contain, such as peppermint or cinnamon, which will tingle when applied, slightly irritate your lips and thus increase the flow of blood to give a bee-stung appearance and added colour. It's basically an inflammatory reaction that works for between two and four hours, but the inflated effect differs from person to person and over-use can make lips very dry.

You will need to change plumpers regularly, too as your lips get used to the added irritant. Also, remember not to kiss anyone when you've just put it on!

★

Be sure to only apply lip plumpers to your lips. If you stray over the lip line, you'll end up with a big red ring around your mouth and people will be offering you a napkin! Freeze 24/7 Plumplips Lip Plumper (freeze247.com) is considered by many to be a pretty perfect plumper.

LINE *Up*

Lip liners can be used effectively to add fullness to lips, but be careful, we don't want Pamela Anderson, circa 90s Baywatch here! As Jerry Seinfeld put it so aptly, 'Where lipstick is concerned, the important thing is not color, but to accept God's final word on where your lips end.' So it's all about subtlety.

★

Add a dash of clear gloss to the upper and lower middle of your lip for a shiny pout.

The first step is to find a nude lip liner that's an exact match to your natural lip line, such as Laura Mercier's Lip Sheer pencil in Natural Lips (lauramercier.com) or Bobbi Brown's Bare or Naked lipliner (both are available at most department stores or online). Now draw a line just outside your natural lip line (don't forget the outer corners) to prevent your lipstick from escaping all over your face like a lunatic from Bedlam and add definition to your mouth. Apply colour with a brush in your usual way and blot with tissue.

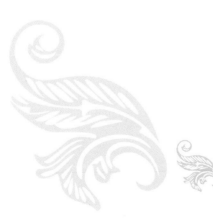

Lauren Hutton shows that you CAN wear dramatic lip colour when older. In 2002 she created her own make-up range 'Good Stuff' for older women saying 'As we age, our faces demand different beauty products and different ways to put them on.' (laurenhutton.com)

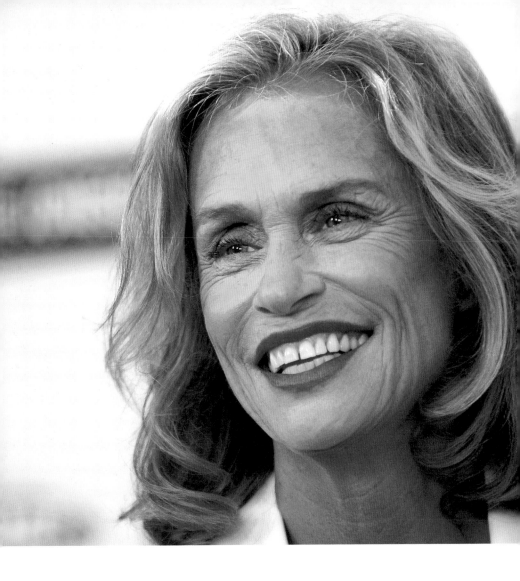

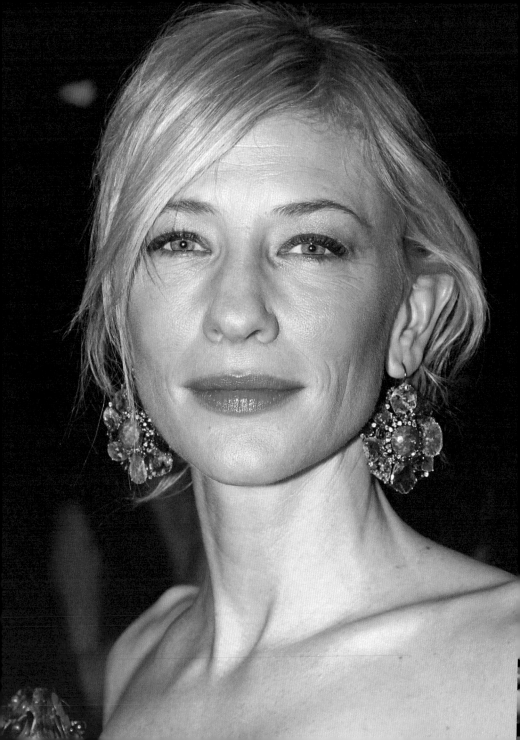

Inside Cate Blanchett's
MAKE-UP BAG

★ **SK II SIGNS EYE MASK** is a cotton pad soaked in moisturizer for treating lines and dark patches under your eyes and targets one of the first areas to show signs of ageing. Cate says it's 'particularly amazing if you pop it in the fridge.' (Available from ski-ii.com – if the price tag scares you, use an old tea bag instead!)

★ **STILA SUN GEL IN BRONZE** – a lightweight gel bronzer that gives her a convincing light tan (beautybay.com).

★ **STILA SHEER COLOR TINTED MOISTURIZER SPF15** in Light to match her dewy skin (hqhair.com).

★ **EAU DU SOIR BY SISLEY** – 'My favourite scent,' says Cate (available at most department stores or online).

Actress Judi Dench famously compared Cate Blanchett's skin to 'a white peach'. The subtle lines in her face show she is not an advocate of Botox but instead recommends 'diligent skin-care'.

'I WOULD RATHER
LOSE A GOOD EARRING
THAN BE CAUGHT
WITHOUT MAKE-UP'

LANA TURNER

LIP SMACKING *Colour*

Actress Carole Lombard once said, 'I live by a man's code, designed to fit a man's world, yet at the same time I never forget that a woman's first job is to choose the right shade of lipstick.' And lo, these are the new lipstick commandments for grown-up glamour!

★ Avoid nude and muted lipsticks – they will make you look a little wraith-like. Low oestrogen levels leach colour from your lips, so have the time of your life with rich hues. Full-on glamour calls for you in the form of fire-engine red (which looks fabulous with grey hair, incidentally) but be warned: you need a mobile, generous mouth for the right effect and a rock-steady hand with a lip brush.

★ If you have thinner lips, still stick with strong colour but change the texture for something softer and replace with a creamier, less intense pigment.

★ Remember that blue-toned reds can be very unforgiving of less-than-white teeth. And on that note, a word of caution – don't be eager to have veneers. It's an invasive procedure that requires continual and excessive aftercare. Red wine, black coffee and green tea are known for their ability to stain the teeth, so a little judicious and subtle teeth whitening might be appropriate. Bear in mind that such procedures can render the teeth excruciatingly sensitive, so anyone who already suffers from sensitive teeth should stick to the whitening toothpastes and a really good toothbrush, such as the Philips Sonicare.

5

HAIR *Dos and Don'ts*

There are lots of cool hairdos about these days, but unfortunately plenty of hair don'ts, too. Why are so many grown-up girls using their hard-earned cash to have the luscious locks of a Russian prisoner-of-war woven onto their own heads? Ratty hair extensions are a crime against hair – they should be the ones thrown in the gulag!

To me, it's unbelievable that we have become so retrospective in our attitude to hair. Britney Spears and Paris Hilton copy their Edwardian ancestors by adding fake pieces of someone else's hair into their own over-processed hairdos. In the early 1900s, women did exactly the same, using fiddly postiches to build up the bulk. But in 1909, women didn't have the vote, HRT or Christian Louboutin, so why would we want the same hair?

Whatever your age, the right cut and colour works wonders and should be chosen on the basis of bone structure, lifestyle and suitability – not the amount you can spend on hair pieces and bleach! As Hubert de Givenchy once said, 'Hair style is the final tip-off whether or not a woman really knows herself' – and he should know because he dressed Audrey Hepburn!

'THE THING ABOUT DOING
ANYTHING ARTIFICIAL TO
YOUR HAIR IS THAT YOU H
AVE TO LOOK AFTER IT. SO
YOU'RE ALWAYS VULNERABLE
TO THE WEATHER AND TIME.'

FRANCESCA ANNIS

BLONDE *is the New Grey*

On the path to karmic bliss, there are many potholes to trip over, but eventually comes the realization that the best enlightenment you can attain is on your own head. As Katie Price slowly morphs into Michael Jackson – same tattooed eyebrows, thickly slick lipsticked lips and jet-black bri-nylon hair – grown-up girls should turn away with a shudder and follow these true glamour rules:

RULE NUMBER ONE: GROW UP, GO LIGHTER

Your hair and skin become paler over time because the melanin in your body is not being produced quite so efficiently as in your twenties, and melanin is what gives hair and skin its colour. Edward Darley, one of the world's top colourists and UK Colour Director at Sassoon, explains, 'There's actually no such thing as grey hair, grey hair is white hair mixed with your natural colour. Your hair has gone white because melanin produces the colour and this is a process that can begin really early on – I had my first grey hair at 14! I have very dark hair so it was more noticeable – you might not notice it in blonde hair for years!'

Girls with grown-up glamour should never, under any circumstances, enter the dark side: it's more ageing and it doesn't suit paler skin. What's more, you'll begin to look like a Gothic freak in a German Expressionist art-house movie. And you don't want crazy carousel music accompanying you wherever you go.

Cyd Charisse, Liza Minnelli and Cher have all hung onto their black hair (Cyd since since the fifties) and they look positively voodoo. So no bad juju for you! Cher, quite frankly, looks even more like a drag queen than the drag queens playing her.

Very dark hair also requires an incredible amount of upkeep, as the re-growth really shows. Edward Darley says: 'You can't have it done too often as your hair will get darker and darker where the tint overlaps, while the re-growth will remain lighter. The dark tinted hair next to the lighter re-growth will make you look as if your wig is slipping off.' If you must persist with this madness, the optimum redo time on a tint is four to six weeks. If the re-growth looks too horrific in the meantime, use hair mascara on the lighter areas.

RULE NUMBER TWO: GO WARMER

Warm tones such as chestnut brown, copper or gold give a sense of heat and if one is added to another, the warmth is increased or decreased, depending on the combination. Warm tones maximize light reflection to give a healthy, glossy sheen to the hair and can also be used to create a sense of movement in a haircut. Stars who have successfully rung this warmer change with their hair colour include the original peroxide punk Debbie Harry, who has now gone for a darker, subtler blonde. Madonna, a bleached boy toy in the eighties, now has hair coloured a soft, multi-tonal golden look that whispers, rather than screams blonde appeal. Julie Christie

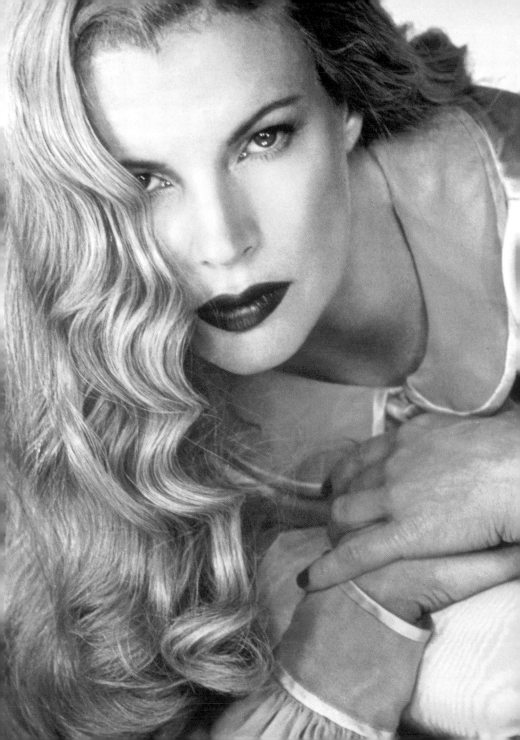

in *Dr Zhivago* (1965) was ice-blonde to match the scenery, while Kim Basinger appeared in *L.A. Confidential* (1997) as an arctic-cool film noir bombshell. Today, both have a softer, more naturally highlighted look in a blend of several tones, including grey. Many heroines of chic prefer to softly camouflage the grey in their hair rather than trying to expunge it altogether. They know that if you stay white-blonde for too long, then at some point you'll begin to look a bit past your sell-by date… Won't you, Pammy Anderson?

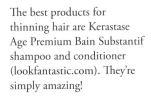

The best products for thinning hair are Kerastase Age Premium Bain Substantif shampoo and conditioner (lookfantastic.com). They're simply amazing!

RULE NUMBER THREE: DON'T STICK IN NO MAN'S LAND

The absolute worst colour that you can have is neither blonde nor brown but looks more like a kind of khaki green – I call it the 'Margaret Thatcher'. The woman who opts for this flat cold colour loves a bring-and-buy sale, is obsessed with kitchen roll and Angela Rippon, and is probably brown naturally. She's followed the lighter rule, but forgotten to add the warmth. So, make the break from brown: don't hang in a mid-colour, take the plunge and go full-on golden blonde.

RULE NUMBER FOUR: NO HOMEGROWN

OK, it's eco, but don't use henna – it only disguises white hair the first few times that you apply it. After that, you'll find that as your hair gets whiter it will turn a lighter orange. Feel free to eat organic vegetables, but don't look like one!

When Kim Basinger played a vamp in *L.A. Confidential* (1997) the ice cold Forties style hairdo fitted the part. Ten years plus later her blonde hair is softer, more natural-looking and perfectly suited to an older skin tone.

RULE NUMBER FIVE: FUNK OFF!

Do not ask your hairdresser for anything 'funky' – in using the word, you become bum-clenchingly embarrassing. Can you remember when your dad kept saying 'groovy' when it was way past its sell-by date? By 'funky', I mean having a little flamingo pink or ultra-violet applied to your hair to 'jazz it up' a bit. Often, this shameful feeling overcomes us at Christmas just before the office party; like similar, dodgy ideas, it should be left to reside in the cobwebbed crypt where it belongs. The problem is not necessarily the colour itself, but the haircut that it's added to. If you take a straightforward do and then 'jazz it up' with a few random streaks, it will immediately look suburban (and thus ageing). Sharon Osbourne always gets it wrong by combining a modern colour with a dull cut – the two must complement each other. Somehow Vivienne Westwood always gets it right because she changes her style regularly and although the colour is a rather flaming orange, it's a warm, flattering tone. Similarly, Pam Hogg's pink works pretty well, too.

RULE NUMBER SIX: WHITE CAN BE SO RIGHT

White hair works brilliantly if the style is modern – a graduated bob on white or grey hair looks amazing. Try to avoid layers and instead go for graphic lines, à la Anna Wintour. Long layered grey hair only makes you look like a roadie for the Grateful Dead!

FOUR FAB *Finishers*

★ **SASSOON DIAMOND POLISH** (sassoon.com) This next-generation serum protects the hair and give it extra shine, especially when using hair straighteners. It has the most amazing buffed effect.

★ **AVEDA SMOOTH INFUSION GLOSSING STRAIGHTENER** (aveda.com) is perfect for those with naturally curly hair that needs a bit of control and shine. This product suits very thick hair. Apply after your hair has been thoroughly towel-dried and then blow dry while using a large brush.

★ **KERASTASE NUTRITIVE VERNIS NUTRI-SCULPT** (luxuryhaircare.co.uk) Long quasi-scientific title for a useful product. Helps smooth dry or chemically treated hair. Whatever your feelings on silicone in other parts of your body – on hair, it works! Silicone closes the hair cuticle and leaves a smooth surface with incredible amounts of increased shine.

★ **REDKEN BLOWN AWAY 09 PROTECTIVE BLOW DRY GEL** (luxuryhaircare.co.uk) acts like a hairspray, serum and gloss in one. Apparently it has 'hair memory' technology so your hair stays in the style that you create, like one of those weird pillows. Hmm… it's a great de-frizzer, though!

Diane von Furstenberg
ON ROLLERS

'I'd rather see a woman with her hair short and nicely manageable than see her walking around at the market with her head packed in jumbo rollers. And I don't think she ought to be in them when her man is home, either. I always wonder what that woman is saving herself for. A woman wouldn't walk out onto the street with a white treatment mask on her face, would she? Well, the rollers are almost the same thing. If your hairdo requires all that time in rollers, I'd say forget it. Being attractive for a few hours some evening is hardly worth being that unattractive all day. Being yourself and being attractive with a man is wonderful, but being downright unattractive with him is foolish.'

THE PERFECT *Blow Dry*

STEP 1 After you have shampooed and conditioned, pat your hair dry with a soft, fluffy towel to remove excess moisture. Hair does not take its final shape until it's almost dry – don't start the process with saturated hair.

STEP 2 A good professional dryer and brush is as important as the product – it will make the blow dry much quicker, as well as far easier! You need a dryer with a range of heat settings, including a cool shot to finish off. Brushes should be half-round, ceramic-tipped designs that control the hair while helping to achieve natural root lift.

STEP 3 Each hair on the head is made up of tiny cuticles that resemble a snake's scales, so in order to create a high shine, it's important that the cuticles lie flat. When working from wet hair to dry, a light straightening lotion will gently smooth and straighten the hair while maintaining its optimum condition. Enhance the effect by keeping the dryer constantly pointed down the shaft of the hair to assist in smoothing the cuticle.

STEP 4 The first stage of the blow dry is called 'wrap drying' and is crucial in achieving natural root movement – it will also help simplify the rest of the finishing process. As the name suggests, the technique is to use the brush to 'wrap' the hair around the head in opposite directions to where it will eventually fall. The dryer, angled toward the root, follows and mirrors the movement of the brush.

STEP 5 When the roots of the hair are 80% dry, start the finishing process on mid-lengths and ends. Take small sections and gently glide the dryer and brush simultaneously down the hair, from root to tip, ensuring that each section is dry before moving on to the next. This technique is known as 'leafing' or 'petalling'.

STEP 6 After the 'leafing' stage is complete, wrap the hair once more. This time, use the dryer on the coolest setting to finish off the blow dry.

STEP 7 Finally, work a small amount of finishing product through to the mid-lengths and ends of your hair to boost shine and bring out the definition of your haircut. It's important not to overload your hair with product – some are very creamy, so a little goes a long way.

Julie Christie treads the red carpet in a perfectly blow-dried bob. The bob should be cut around the mid neck and lightly layered. Use a volumizer and blow out the hair with a round brush.

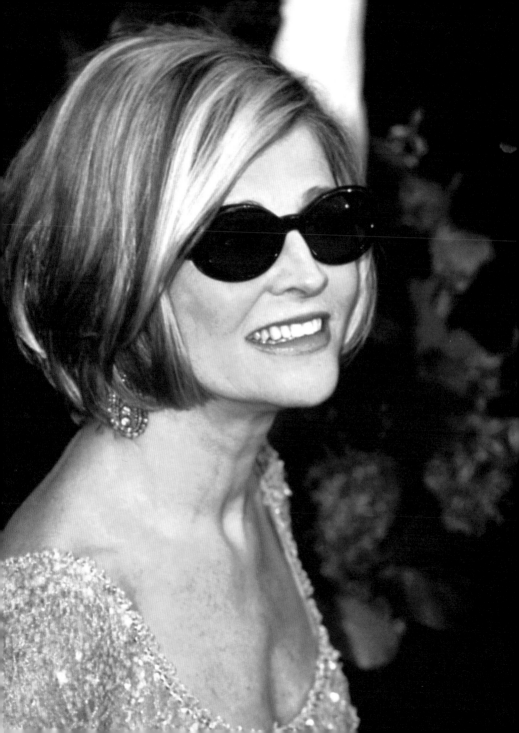

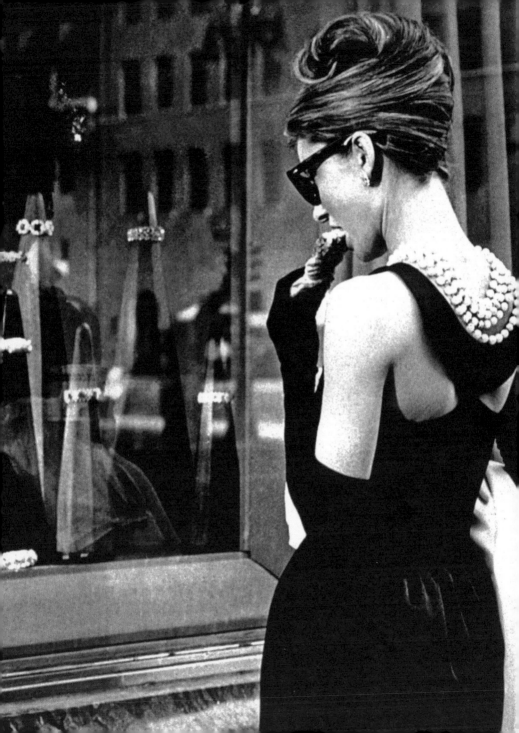

HOW TO GET THE
Audrey Hepburn French Pleat

The most iconic French pleat on celluloid is the one sported by Audrey Hepburn's character, Holly Golightly, in *Breakfast at Tiffany's* (1961). Today celebrated fashionista Daphne Guinness wears it regularly. To get the look perfectly, you need to have a short, choppy fringe. Audrey's fringe is cut unevenly, and then sliced into with the points of the scissors to give it texture. This style requires a bit of commitment, but if you want the authentic look then you'll need to bite the bullet. Here's how:

STEP 1 Put heated rollers through your hair, winding from front to back. This style needs lots of volume to work.

STEP 2 Brush out your hair and backcomb it – you're going big, baby!

STEP 3 Separate your fringe so that it appears mussed up rather than lying in a straight line.

STEP 4 Pull all the hair from one side to the back of your head and pin it in place with hair grips criss-crossed vertically up the middle of the back of your head.

STEP 5 Gather all the remaining hair and twist to form a roll that covers the criss-cross grips. Push grips into the edge of the roll to secure it invisibly. The higher you start the twist, the higher it gets!

STEP 6 Use a firm control hairspray to set.

Audrey Hepburn's French pleat in *Breakfast at Tiffany's* (1961) was given a textured effect with the use of tan blonde highlights on her usually dark brown hair.

Long-haired Ladies, **LISTEN UP**

For many grown-up girls in the twenty-first century, the preoccupation is: when do I cut my hair? It's that old 16/61 problem – you look 16 from behind, but then when you turn round, oops, practically pensionable! There's just something a little icky about having the long blonde hair of a teenager when you're not – a bit like the scene in *She* (1965), the Hammer movie based on H. Rider Haggard's novel, when Ursula Andress morphs from a sex siren into a raddled old hag, or Olivia Hussey in *Lost Horizon* (1973) where the same metamorphosis occurs, this time in Tibet.

HOW TO MAKE LONG HAIR WORK
Long, undressed hair only works if it's worn away from the face – when it's long and dangling, you may think you look like Megan Fox but it's more like Alice Cooper.

★ Hair worn just above the shoulder has more structure and brings out the angles of the face. If it's on the shoulder or below, it pulls the face down.

★ **JERRY HALL**'s locks are getting shorter, though not short enough. Her hair tip is to apply sunflower oil to the ends of your hair and leave overnight to prevent split ends.

★ **MARIE HELVIN** is said never to visit a hairdresser! She looks after her long hair herself: 'I'm very gentle with it, giving myself a treatment once a month. I rub in hot almond oil, wrap my head in a towel and leave it on for as long as possible.' (She's also started tinting it herself and I think it's way too dark!)

★ **MONICA BELLUCCI** can still get away with long hair... but then Monica Bellucci can get away with anything. Miaow!

★ ─────★─────

If your hair isn't long enough to have one high ponytail or it's layered, make two (one slightly higher than the other). Pull the first ponytail over the second to hide it and disguise the band with a barrette.

★ If you want to keep your long hair, wear it in a simple 'updo' like **GRACE KELLY** or **AUDREY HEPBURN**. You can't imagine Audrey with her hair down, can you?

★ **CARLA BRUNI** has hair that dips beyond her shoulders at the back, but she's careful to wear it off her face with a demi-fringe. She rocks a great Hepburnesque coiled French pleat at formal events and is rumoured to use Phytovolume Actif Maximizing Volume Spray (sephora.com), especially formulated for fine and long, limp hair. The product contains keratin amino acids to add body and give roots a lift. You don't get the crunchiness that you can sometimes get with other volumizers, either. Add a light spritz for high volume and style.

HAIRSTYLES OF THE *Great She-Beasts*

Can you imagine these people with a different do?

★ **QUEEN ELIZABETH II** has had same hair style for most of her life. It's almost as if she arrived from the womb with the same cemented do. Her hair is pure anti-fashion, seeming as unassailable the monarchy itself. We seem to be able to cope with a slight change in the hair of royalty as long as it concerns one of the minor royals, such as Zara Phillips, second child of the Princess Royal. Such a change in the British Queen is taboo. Perhaps her fixed appearance makes her subjects feel secure – she remains immutable if she's always set outside the parameters of fashion because she, like her hair, seems to always be there. The magic of Liz's do is that it has come full circle and looks almost good now, so if you're prepared to ride it out like our dear monarch for fifty years and can freeze out stifled giggles, silent laughter and sideways glances from your subjects, go for it!

★ **MARGARET (MAGGIE) THATCHER** has had a complete image overhaul. On gaining power, first as the leader of the Conservative Party and then as British Prime Minister, she wore suits with heavily padded shoulders, a feminized tie in the guise of a pussycat bow, high heels, discreet jewellery and, most significantly, bouffant hair. Her large, heavily set and sprayed style gives the illusion of a hard helmet – as she climbed to power, her hair became larger and larger, as if to have a life of its own. If you have a mad lust for power, mercury for blood and steel in your soul, this look is perfect for you – the rest of us can only stand back and gaze in awe.

★ **LINDA EVANS** has been wearing her long blonde *Dynasty* do since the 1980s. Teamed with power shoulders and Blake Carrington, it has seductive appeal in the brash style of the decade. So too do Kylie's bubble perm, Grace Jones's Cameo cut and Boy George's blusher – we just wouldn't want to be wearing them now!

★ **GOLDIE HAWN** needs to modernize her look. She still has the same hairstyle as when starring in *Private Benjamin* (1980) and almost the same hair as her daughter, Kate Hudson, has today. The before-and-after effect when the two are together is a little disconcerting.

★ **DONATELLA VERSACE** – bleached blonde hair, fake-and-bake tan, puffed-up pucker… Has she been taking beauty tips from a mortician?

★ **LIZA MINNELLI** gave the performance of her career in 1972 as Sally Bowles, dancer at Berlin's Kit Kat Club in the film *Cabaret*. She is said to have designed her own hair and make-up for the film and as an evocation of decadent Weimar it was faultless. Splayed over a chair vampishly crooning Bye Bye Mein Herr it should have been Bye Bye My Hair as she's still sporting the same jet black crop with Twenties kiss curl.

★ **DOLLY PARTON** Bright, back-combed, bri-nylon blonde. I just think it's weird when a woman's hair is taller than she is.

Britt Ekland
ON UP-DOS

'Keep it simple. Rather than contorting your hair into the traditional confines of the French pleat, try this. Bend over, brush all your hair forward and just grab it into a bunch at the edge of your forehead. Catch it in an elastic band, stand up and twirl your hair around into a little knot. Don't worry about the back bits falling loose – that just gives you a softer, prettier profile. If this doesn't happen naturally, you can take a comb or use your fingers to pull a couple of little tendrils around your face. Don't pull the bun too tight, whatever you do. Most women look better with a softer line, and in my case it has the added advantage of hiding my ears.'

WAXING *Lyrical*

If you are prepared to remove one of the prime signs of your sexual maturity, and publicly put yourself in a position normally reserved for athletic bedroom activity, by all means go for a Brazilian wax. It's not like a bikini wax, where you just shift your knickers about a bit – this will leave you with a landing strip in the front and nothing else. Be prepared to strip from the waist down, then lie down on your back while another woman peers at your lady-garden, sprinkles baby powder all over it and then applies warm wax. She'll slap your thigh to divert you, then rip! Yoweeeee! The pain is unbearable, you will throb (and not in a good way), there will be itching as it grows back – and don't mention the 5 o'clock shadow.

Jerry Hall broke a taboo when she said, '*When you get older, your ears get big and flappy – no one ever tells you that. Oh, and you get hair in weird places.*' Female facial hair! It's one of the consequences of getting older because as oestrogen levels decline and testosterone takes over, hair begins to sprout unexpectedly – most notably on the chin and (gulp) big toe. The odd bristle is easy, just pluck it out. The real problem is facial fuzz on the upper lip and around the jaw. Facial depilatory creams are cheap and painless and work by dissolving hair at the base of the follicle but make sure you do a patch test first as they can sometimes irritate sensitive skin. The Bellabe has its fans too, a bit of kit that works on the principle of threading and with practice can be very effective (amazon.com).

6

THE GROWN-UP
Glamour Awards

It's now time to focus the spotlight on some of our most glamorous grown-ups, whether it's because of their beauty, charm, personality, rebellious acts or just plain good humour. On and off the red carpet these women are heroines and for this we celebrate them. As glamorous grown-ups ourselves, we appreciate fabulousness, wherever and however it appears.

For some of us, laurel wreaths and badges of honour may come a little later in life: Doris Lessing received the Nobel Prize for Literature at the age of 88; Anna Mary Robertson a.k.a. Grandma Moses, one of America's most popular artists, sold her first painting at the age of 78, and Katharine Hepburn won a Best Actress Oscar for *Guess Who's Coming to Dinner* in her 60th year. Mary Wesley's first novel, *Jumping the Queue*, was published when she was 70 and the Canadian Jeannie Reiman was still competing in car racing at a sprightly 90. Quite rightly, these achievements should be lauded and they have also spurred those of us in a little less highbrow world to give out some accolades of our own – this time in the field of grown-up glamour. Our feminist sensibilities may baulk a little at singling out just one aspect of these fabulous older women, rather than concentrating on the whole package, but we want to have something achievable to aim for!

'IT'S THE CRÈME DE LA CRÈME OF BULLSHIT.'

HELEN MIRREN ON THE ACADEMY AWARDS

HELEN MIRREN'S
Bikini

Hitting 40 can bring on extremes of decision-making: less kebabs, more kiwifruit; detox over retox (hold that third Kir Royale) and no more bikinis on the beach. But on 16 July 2008, only a few days away from her 63rd birthday, A-list goddess Helen Mirren was papped in Puglia on the southernmost tip of Italy in a very fetching bright red, low-rise two-piece. To celebrate winning an Oscar for Best Actress, she had purchased a 500-year-old castle complete with its own vineyard in nearby Lecce for £680,000 in 2007. (How one sentence can sum up a glamorous grown-up's life!)

Mirren's bikini appearance made headlines around the world – she was voluptuous yet toned; her breasts full but not fake; and most importantly, Dame Helen looked fabulous without any need for airbrushing or the dreaded thigh-disguising sarong! Granted she hasn't had any kids, which helps with her enviably flat stomach, and she was sucking it in as her husband Taylor Hackford took a photo – but even so… It was one of those few and far between media images: a woman with a real body, not some malnourished double-zero size celeb with a pair of surgically enhanced breasts that could take your eye out.

Posing in the sun, white-haired and a little wrinkled, Mirren displayed a complete lack of the paralysing self-criticism that befalls many of us after a certain age, although she minimized the impact that her photo had, saying: 'It was pure luck, honestly. I swear to you, I do not look like that. I look at that picture and say, "God, I wish I looked like that!" but in reality I don't – I just carry on my own sweet way. I learned fairly early in my life that you are two things – you are what other people see you as being, and you are what you see yourself as being, and you will never see what other people see. You will never see what I'm looking at because I'm looking at you, and you will never see yourself as I see you, in your whole life. You are two people for the whole of your life and I came to terms with that a long time ago, so I let people get on with it. I'm just who I am, and I deal with the person that I know I am.'

AFTERWORD

The pictures were not set up, but strategically planned by photographer Mario Brenna, who had been scouting local beaches for signs of the A-list star. There were 23 shots in all, and it's important to stress that the most flattering were chosen. As the syndicator who parlayed the shots out to the media, Jason Fraser, said: 'I couldn't see the point in syndicating a photo of a woman sat down on a beach, leaning forward and putting sun cream on. If these shots had been set up, their charisma would have been diminished. Helen Mirren is stunning enough to not need to prepare herself for a planned photo.'

Interestingly, it was pure luck that caused the photos to surface at all, their value only increased by a shortage of other celeb pictures at the start of the summer – and apparently because Mirren was wearing a red bikini rather than a black one that made all the difference. Industry sources say the images fetched £100,000.

KATHLEEN TURNER'S
Voice

'You aren't too smart, are you? I like that in a man.' With that one provocative line delivered in a distinctive smoky tone, we were introduced to Kathleen Turner in the steamy film noir of 1981, *Body Heat*. Voices are incredibly important. How many times have you been drawn to someone, but when they open their mouth the illusion is shattered? A prime example is David Beckham. Conversely we can be mesmerized by a voice: Orson Welles' perfect intonation; Grace Kelly's patrician tone, Ellen Barkin's huskiness and Maggie Smith's prim eccentricity – where would they be without their dulcet tones?

———— ★ ————

If you want a voice like Kathleen Turner's, take a look at Arthur Lessac's voice production training (lessacinstitute.com). Workshops are held all around the world. One of his strangest exercises, as followed by Kathleen, is to remove the little eraser from the end of a pencil and put it in the back of your mouth between your teeth. This apparently teaches you to stretch your mouth muscles and helps to add more timbre to your voice.

Turner believes we all have the potential to improve our voices and thus, their effectiveness: 'It seems to me that, particularly for women, having a good vocal presence completes you. I mean, what does it matter what you look like if people cringe when you open your mouth?' Like our fingerprints, our voices are unique – and her advice? Training. 'I meet women who look very glamorous – they've got about five thou on the hoof, right? The hair, the clothes, the jewellery… And then they open their mouth and their voice is so annoying and off-putting. Why don't they take the amount they spent on one outfit and go get voice lessons?'

MICHELLE OBAMA'S *Arms*

A magic moment – a fortysomething Michelle Obama steps into the global spotlight in 2009, sporting a sleeveless shift from which emerge the most perfectly toned and sculpted arms – now her A-list trademark. Barack's policies be damned, his wife's arms have inspired more headlines! The new Mrs O has daily workouts with personal trainer Cornell McClellan that include reps of tricep pushdowns using a pulley for resistance and hammer curls with weights; the good news is that the arm exercises are said to take only nine minutes. The bad news is that she combines them with a 5.30am fitness regime of kickboxing, weight training and skipping, plus a healthy eating regime.

Let's just aim for the arms, hey? So dust off your dumbbells and have a go! Your rear upper arms (a.k.a. bingo wings) are, of course, your triceps, the name for the muscle that goes down the back of your arm. Triceps go floppy because they are non-weight-bearing muscles – to improve matters you need to tone 'em up by giving them a good workout. The following exercises are simple, effective and you don't need to shell out for a personal trainer like Michelle – just a little self-motivation.

Dust Off Your Dumbbells!

EXERCISE 1

You can do this one either standing or sitting.

1 Keep your back straight at all times. Now take a dumbbell in each hand (you can use a bag of sugar instead but it must be the finest muscovado – joke!).

2 With arms outstretched, raise them to shoulder height; hold for ten seconds before bringing them back down to waist height.

EXERCISE 2

Start by doing ten of these exercises each day, then add light weights.

1 Hold your arms out to the sides of your body so they are level with your shoulders. With your fingers pointed, make small circles. Do this backwards and forwards.

2 Now hold your hands out level with your shoulders so the palms are facing upwards. With small movements, lift your arms up and down. Repeat the action with your palms facing downwards.

EXERCISE 3

Wear light wrist weights when you're doing the cleaning. Whaddya mean, you don't do cleaning? Writer and self-confessed 'stately homo of England' Quentin Crisp once advised that you should leave the dust in your home undisturbed: 'I have a message of hope for the housewives of England. After four years it doesn't get any worse.'

Michelle Obama says, 'Women in particular need to keep an eye on their physical and mental health, because if we're scurrying to and from appointments and errands, we don't have a lot of time to take care of ourselves. We need to do a better job of putting ourselves higher on our own "to do" list.'

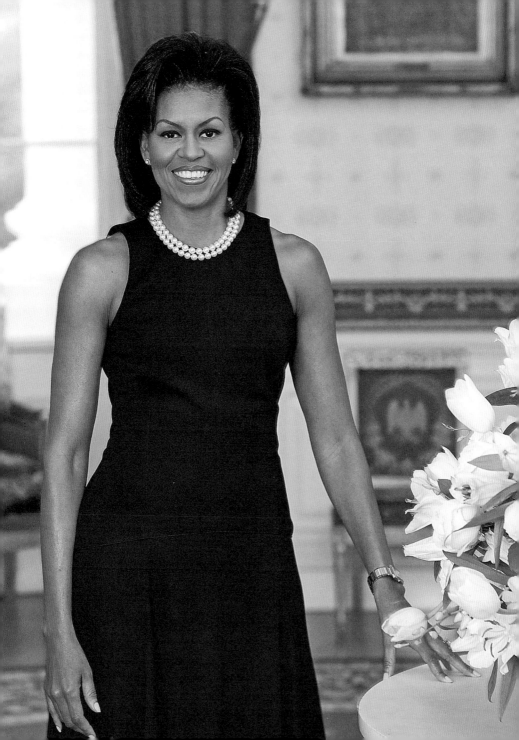

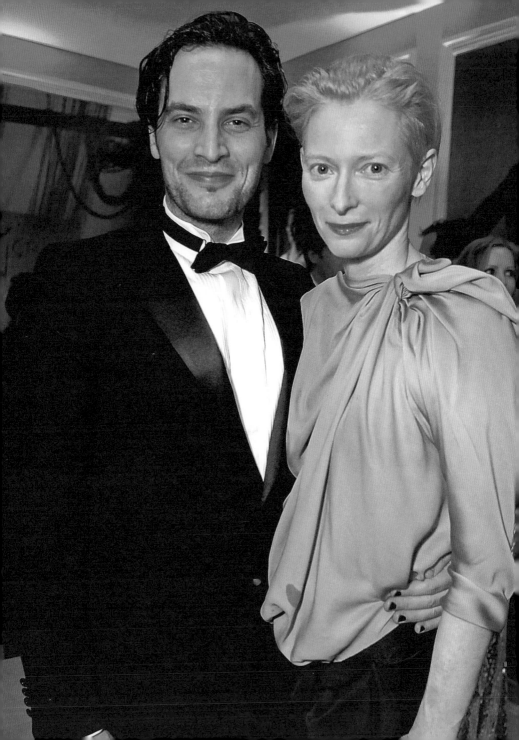

For Successfully Juggling a Bohemian Love Life
TILDA SWINTON

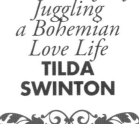

Milky-white skin, Titian hair and constantly bedecked in the most avant-garde couture, risk-taking actress Tilda Swinton has been a mesmerizing red-carpet presence throughout her fifty years on the planet.

And her love life is no less gripping as she manages to juggle two men. Long-term love, and father of her twins Xavier and Honor, is the renowned  Scottish artist John Byrne, who is more than twenty years older than her. Then there's the consort to her Narnian Ice Queen, Sandro Kopp, an artist who, rather neatly, is almost twenty years younger – they met when he was playing a centaur in *The Lion, the Witch and the Wardrobe* (2005).

According to Tilda, it's an arrangement that works very well: '*John and I live with our children and Sandro is sometimes here with us, and we travel the world together. We are all a family.*'

Tilda, we salute you!

Tilda Swinton accompanied by her boyfriend Sandro Kopp, part of a bohemian ménage that includes her husband, artist John Byrne and father of their twins. 'The arrangement is just so sane' says Tilda.

TALLULAH BANKHEAD'S *Wit*

Playwright Tennessee Williams called her the result of the fantastic crossbreeding of a moth and a tiger and she was reputedly the inspiration for Cruella de Vil in the film *101 Dalmatians*. Five foot three inches tall, movie star Tallulah Bankhead's trademark was her rasping sandpaper voice and mordant wit. A drunken bisexual rebel, who died at 65. Despite an illustrious stage career, she had only one filmic hit to her name: Alfred Hitchcock's *Lifeboat* of 1944. However, Tallulah has bestowed a legacy of pithy bons mots and razor-sharp repartee on us grown-up girls.

She enjoyed affairs with many of the Hollywood greats, including Marlene Dietrich, who had an adjoining dressing room in the 1930s, where they would flirt over copious flutes of champagne. Dietrich was well known for dusting her hair with gold to subtly catch the glint of the studio lights on set. On more than one instance Tallulah applied it to her nether regions and would then open the door to unsuspecting passers-by, giving them, quite literally, a Sapphic flash. '*Whaddya think I've just been doing, Daaahling?*' she drawled.

TALLULAH ON BAD HABITS
'I'm as pure as driven slush.'

'Daddy warned me about men and alcohol but he never warned me about women and cocaine.'

'Cocaine isn't habit forming. I should know, I've been using it for years.'

'A frozen daiquiri of a scorching afternoon is soothing. It makes living more tolerable.'

TALLULAH ON SEX
'I'll come and make love to you at 5 o'clock. If I'm late, start without me.'

On seeing a lover for the first time in many years: 'I thought I told you to wait in the car.'

TALLULAH ON LIFE
'I'd rather be strongly wrong than weakly right.'

'If I had to live my life again I'd make the same mistakes – only sooner.'

'They used to shoot Shirley Temple through gauze. They should shoot me through linoleum.'

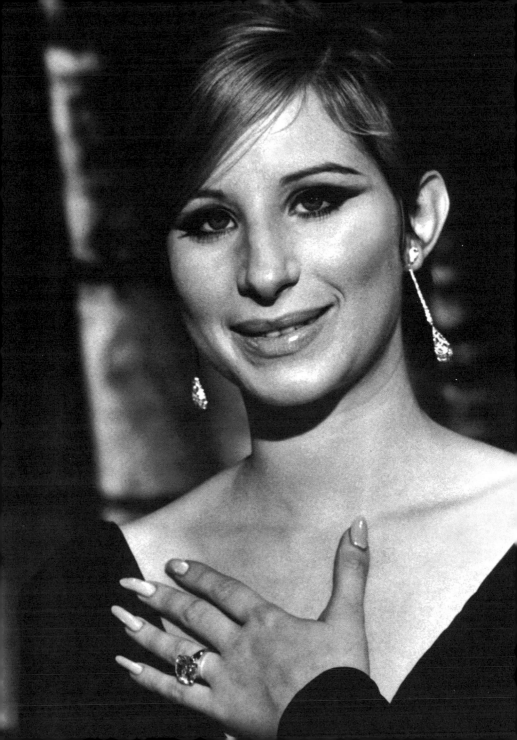

And Special Mentions Go To…

BARBRA STREISAND'S *Nails*

Nail moments captured on celluloid don't happen too often (save the faux orgasmic scratching down the back in a soft-focus Sixties sex scene). Of course, there's the sequence in *The Women* (1939) when Norma Shearer finds out about her husband's cheatin' ways through her manicurist, who has been glossing another woman's nails in her man's pet colour, the aptly named Jungle Red. But it's Barbra Streisand's nails that have stuck out (literally) over her long and rather chequered movie career.

Who can forget the flashy Sixties manicure that made the divine film *Funny Girl* (1968), supposedly set in the 1910s, so historically inaccurate? Barbra's histrionic nail baring dominates practically every scene. Or *The Main Event* (1979), where lingering close-ups make the most of her glossy long talons? But the most outstanding nail shots in the singer's career come in *The Prince of Tides* (1991), where she rocks a serious French polish and started a global trend for the manicure that continues today.

Why the nails? According to Streisand, this was a form of rebellion: '*Mum said, "You've got to study typing. That's what you're going to do with your life." I grew my fingernails long so I couldn't study typing. To this day, I can't type – I write everything in longhand.*'

Barbra Streisand is said to have a manicure every day. For healthy nails for less cash, celebrity manicurist Jessica Vartoughian says, 'Tap fingers regularly on a hard surface – nails are nourished by blood flow.'

NAIL FACTS

★ **BARBRA STREISAND** loves OPI's Bogota Blackberry (opi.com) so much that she had her car, a Ford Expedition, painted in exactly the same shade to match her toenail polish.

★ When questioned by the police in relation to a possible weapons charge against her boyfriend P Diddy, **JENNIFER LOPEZ** reputedly asked the officer to get her some cuticle cream!

★ **JOAN CRAWFORD** once said that you should match your nails to the amount of make-up you wear: '*Exotic nails and an unsophisticated complexion do not go together.*'

NAIL TIPS FOR GLAMOROUS GROWN-UPS

More than any other part of the body, hands reveal the passing of time, so if you're not happy with yours, then it might be best to deflect attention from them rather than flash your digits emblazoned with Chanel's 407 Jade. Start applying sunscreen to them to prevent the formation of age spots, too.

★ Keep nails short and neutral. Red lacquered claws filed to a point are an instantly ageing look.

★ Avoid fake nails; they require a lot of upkeep and you'll seem less glamorous grown-up, more reject from The Hills.

★ Squared-off French manicured nails with thick white tips look cheap. Go for a natural, slightly more rounded shape with thinly applied off-white tips.

★ Absolutely no nail art and no glitter. Ever.

For Glamour in Extreme Circumstances
SHEILA LEGGE

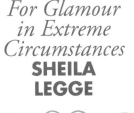

The International Surrealist Exhibition was held in London in 1936 at the New Burlington Galleries. At the first night opening the crush was so great that traffic in Piccadilly was left in gridlock and over the next three weeks 40,000 people visited, inspired in no small part by the antics of artist Salvador Dalí, who famously gave an address while sporting a deep-sea diving suit. He began to suffocate until he was mercifully extracted with a spanner.

The highlight of the show was a living sculpture by Dalí entitled 'The Phantom of Sex Appeal', for which the artist Sheila Legge solemnly glided through the crowded gallery in a skin-tight white satin gown, her head encased in a wire cage covered in pink paper rosebuds, a female mannequin's leg in her hand (although Dalí had insisted on a pork chop).

'That get-up must be very hot,' whispered one bystander.

'Very!' murmured Legge.

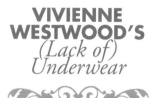

VIVIENNE WESTWOOD'S *(Lack of) Underwear*

In 1992, at the age of 51, Vivienne Westwood attended Buckingham Palace to collect her OBE from HM the Queen. After the ceremony a demurely dressed Westwood twirled in the courtyard for photographers and her full-circle skirt flew up to reveal that she was wearing no knickers under a pair of rather suburban beige tights – and displayed a pair of the most amazing legs! Cue outrage…

In 2006, she was at it again. After having been made a Dame, she unabashedly disclosed that she was knickerless at Buck House for the second time in her career, adding: 'Don't ask: it's the same answer, I don't wear them with dresses. When I'm wearing trousers I might – my husband's silk boxers.'

Her outfit again was delicious: a black dress with net stole smothered in campaign badges, a matching black hat perched on the back of her head of vivid orange hair plus a pair of tiny pagan horns attached by a wire – worn as a calling card for what she called 'a new renaissance' as 'we don't have culture'. Looking like a magical mix of urban Fifties housewife and cool jungle guerrilla, Westwood described her ensemble as a reflection of 'my political feeling. I'm supposed to be a bit like a Che Guevara with my cap, this kind of jungle net and a badge for my Active Resistance to Propaganda campaign.' If you're interested in Viv's politics, learn more by visiting activeresistance.co.uk/index1.html.

For Being Funny, Fat and Fabulous
SHELLEY WINTERS

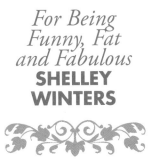

Shelley Winters was an old-school bombshell, described by Frank Sinatra as 'a bow-legged bitch of a blonde' who had a long Hollywood career that started in the Fifties. Round-faced, big bosomed and quite frankly, fat (UK size 20 in *The Poseidon Adventure* of 1972), she shrugged off intimations that she should lose weight by saying, 'I'm not overweight – I'm just nine inches too short.'

An infamous seductress, her list of conquests included Marlon Brando, whom she described as 'sexual lightning', Sean Connery (when he was hot rather than grumpy), Robert De Niro, Albert Finney, Burt Lancaster, Clark Gable, Errol Flynn – and most surprising of all, Farley Granger (he didn't normally stray on that side of the fence!). When a sozzled Dylan Thomas told her at a Hollywood bash that he had come to Tinseltown 'to touch the titties of a beautiful blonde starlet and to meet Charlie Chaplin,' she instantly proffered her pneumatic bosom. Later in life she admitted, '*Now that I'm 60, I'm veering towards respectability. I have bursts of being a lady, but it doesn't last long!*'

For Subtle Art of Persuasion
JOANNA LUMLEY

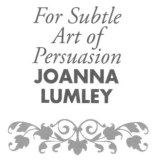

In 2007, actress Joanna Lumley (61 at the time) was engaged in an interview in a theatre bar when a gunman interrupted her spiel as his weapon clattered to the floor. Calmly she walked over, sat next to him and engaged him in charming conversation until the police arrived.

Lumley is a goddess – literally. In 2008, she fronted a campaign to give all Gurkha veterans who served in the British Army before 1997 the right to settle in Britain. Following this success, the people of Nepal declared Joanna Lumley a goddess. Grown-up girls can learn some serious lessons from this example, as the campaign was won not through brute force or fierce intellect, but persuasion. One journalist described her press briefings and committee hearings as 'organized drools', with the politicians 'rolling on their backs like puppy-dogs to have their tummies tickled'.

HOW TO PERSUADE LUMLEY-STYLE

★ 'Water is strong and a river running down, if you dam it, will break the dam. So find a way round. And if you can find a way round, it's usually much better and people don't get hurt. And people don't lose face, which is terribly important. But if a change of mind can take place in their own minds, rather than being forced to it – I think it's the best way to do anything.'

★ 'I don't lose my temper. I've governed myself not to mind about things. I have no road rage or anything like that because it's life shortening and also there's no need for it, it uses up energy. I don't mind not eating, or sitting in the bad part of a restaurant or being snubbed, it doesn't really matter to me very much.'

★ 'I hate the hand that comes out of a car and just drops litter in the street. I hate that! For some reason it just fills me with fury. It's just utter laziness, lack of interest in other people, lack of interest in the planet, in the hedgehog who might eat the plastic bag – it's a lack of concern. I would package it up and say, "I believe you dropped this." And if they were horrid, I would think of a different way of dealing with it.'

AND JUST TO SHOW THE WOMAN REALLY IS A SAINT...

'In service stations on big motorways I always clean up the ladies loo. I pick up all the bits of hankies, I tidy up the bins, I get using the towels, I clean the tops, I shut the doors; I pull the plugs because people live like animals. And surely if it looks nice, people won't go on making it look so bad?'

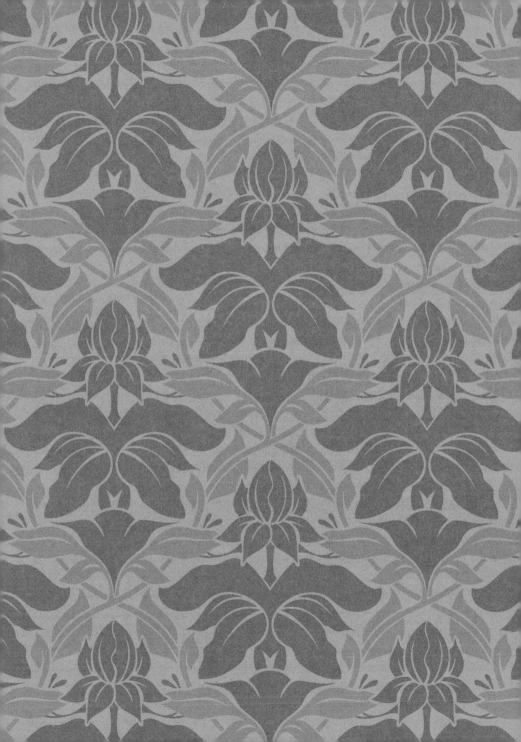

7

Joining the **JET SET**

I have a motto when it comes to a holiday – No-Frills equals No-Thrills. For me, the days of InterRailing across Europe, sleeping on the roof of a Greek pension or camping in a sodden field in the Lakes are long gone. Now I want a holiday with a bit of va va voom or I'd rather stay home, watch re-runs of *Dynasty* and channel Alexis Colby.

Jackie O loved a vacation, seeing it as the chance to experience something new and culturally authentic – as she put it: 'I know that to visit Seville and not ride horseback at the fair is equal to not coming at all!' And in 1968, while at the Yucatan peninsula, her travel companion noted: 'She wasn't content just to see the Mayan ruins by daytime – she also insisted on seeing them by moonlight, on horseback, to get the feeling of the way it was the day before yesterday. And once she tossed herself into a pool near the ruins with all her clothes on.' (I must confess Jackie's approach is not necessarily my own and the closest I have been is the donkey ride from Santorini Port up to my boutique hotel!)

GETAWAYS *with Grown-Up Glamour*

It shouldn't be all work, work, work for us grown-up girls: every now and again we need to re-charge our batteries on a suitably glamorous break. As Marlene Dietrich once said, *'If you can manage to have ice-cold Dom Perignon in a beautiful glass on the terrace of a Paris restaurant looking onto trees in a midday autumn sun you will feel like the most luxurious grown-up in the world.'*

Not for us the teeming Irish taverns of Tenerife or the sweltering golf courses of the Algarve – we sophisticates need something a little more elegant. Movie stars used to know how to have a weekend away – Ava Gardner ran off to Madrid at the drop of a matador's hat, Brigitte Bardot was never out of her gingham bikini in St Tropez, and Liz Taylor had to be prised from Portofino to get on set. Budget airlines and package tours be damned: follow in the footsteps of those who know how and have the time of your life!

LOS ANGELES *Kim Novak Style*

Kim Novak was once a hat-check-girl-turned-model from Chicago, who hung out in the City of Angels after touring the country as Miss Deepfreeze to publicize a refrigerator company. In the early Fifties she was signed up by Columbia's Harry Coen as a Marilyn Monroe lookalike and by 1957 she had become a major box-office star, featuring on the cover of *Time Magazine*. She had a haunting, melancholic quality that drew men to her with almost a siren's call, including Frank Sinatra, Cary Grant and Sammy Davis Jr. Fearing a public backlash over this particular relationship, Coen called on the Mafia hit men to force Davis into a shotgun wedding with a Vegas showgirl. Today Novak is nearly 80 and spends her time painting on a ranch in California.

In LaLa Land you'll find that you have to get a cab everywhere! The city is huge, humid and sprawling with no discernible centre and no one walks – the residents will stare at you with curiosity if you do. If you've never been there before you must visit Grauman's Chinese Theatre on Hollywood Boulevard, which opened in 1927. Fights broke out as fans tried to catch a glimpse of their favourite stars – and the Art-Deco LA Union Station.

For the full Fifties' experience, start with lunch in **CANTER'S DELI** at 491 Fairfax Avenue, reputedly a favourite haunt of Kim's as well as odd couple Marilyn Monroe and playwright Arthur Miller. Have a hot pastrami sandwich or chicken matzoth ball soup. Or drive to **PINK'S HOTDOG STAND** on 709 North La Brea Ave and munch on a chilli dog. Pink's proximity to Paramount Pictures has made it legendary in Hollywood and it harks back to the days when kids with dreams used to pin their headshots and phone numbers on the walls in the hope of being discovered. Orson Welles still holds the record for eating the most hot dogs in one sitting – 18! It's also the spot where Sean Penn proposed to Madonna and Bruce Willis to Demi Moore.

For pre-dinner drinks, try **BOARDNER'S BAR** (1652 N. Cherokee Ave) – a snug, voluptuously curving bar, neon-lit and steeped in Hollywood history, or the **FORMOSA** (7156 Santa Monica Blvd), which opened in 1934 and is festooned with faded and autographed photos of its star-studded patrons. Then eat enchiladas tapatias and check the ambience at **LUCY'S EL ADOBE** Mexican restaurant at 5536 Melrose Ave, an old school studio hang-out, or **EL COYOTE** (7312 Beverly Boulevard), purveyor of Mexican food to such stars as Loretta Young, John Wayne, Princess Grace and Prince Rainier of Monaco since 1930. If you don't like hot tamales and margaritas (what's wrong with you?), try the classic Italian **MICELI'S RESTAURANT** at 1646 Las Palmas Avenue. And

FOR ARMCHAIR TRAVELLERS

WATCH *Strangers When We Meet* (1960): Kim Novak and Kirk Douglas in an amazing study of suburban infidelity filmed on location in Brentwood, Malibu and Beverly Hills.

READ *The Day of The Locust* by Nathaniel West (1939), an ironic Depression-era novel that examines a motley group of Hollywood hangers-on.

if you're a fan of *Mad Men* (and who isn't?), you must go to **MUSSO & FRANK'S** at 6667 Hollywood Boulevard, which starred in Season 1, Episode 7. Open since 1919, this dimly lit film noir style restaurant (Raymond Chandler wrote *The Big Sleep* here) has served Greta Garbo, Claudette Colbert and Bette Davis. The walls are wood-panelled, the booths upholstered in the same shade of leather as the waiters' jackets and you can get shrimp cocktails and oyster pie as well as a standard steak.

Stay at the **SUNSET TOWER HOTEL** (sunsettowerhotel.com), a beautiful example of Art-Deco architecture on the fabled Sunset Boulevard that was originally a block of luxury apartments. Residents included Greta Garbo, Mae West, Carole Lombard and John Wayne, who kept a pet cow on his balcony so that guests could have fresh milk with their coffee. Eccentric millionaire Howard Hughes housed several of his mistresses there and a snap-brimmed Frank Sinatra had a bachelor pad where he proposed to Ava Gardner as she drunkenly draped herself over his balcony. In the Seventies Iggy Pop used to dive from his apartment window straight into the pool – his drug use was such that he would miss and was rushed to hospital a couple of times a month. Sadly, the tower fell into disrepair in the Eighties until it was converted into a lovely luxury hotel.

Kim Novak with Marlon Brando at a Los Angeles awards dinner. So much of old Hollywood has disappeared, but for info on what's left and how to find it go to laconservancy. org, who are helping curate the city.

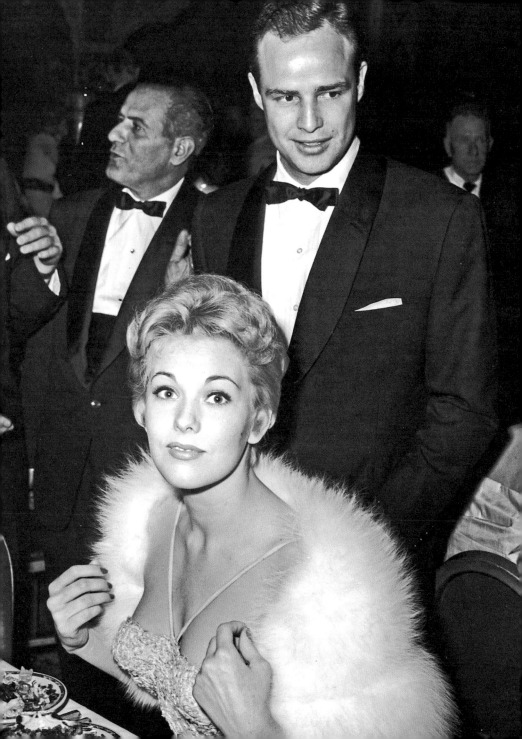

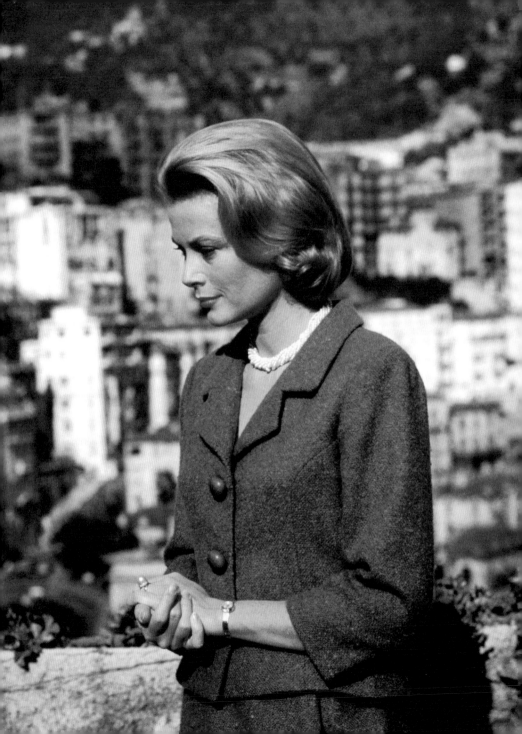

MONTE CARLO *Grace Kelly Style*

In the divine *Rebecca* (1940), starring the gorgeously delicate Joan Fontaine, the action starts when our heroine meets Maxim de Winter, played by a sexy and saturnine Laurence Olivier, while sitting in the lobby of the Hotel de Paris in Monte Carlo. She is a paid companion to the snippy and diamond-emblazoned socialite Edythe Van Hopper, who is abstracted and angry as her usual set aren't around. Maxim asks what she thinks of the area, to which she replies, 'Artificial.' Ms Van Hopper harrumphs the immortal lines, **'*Most girls would give their eyes for the chance to see Monte.*'** And it's true, especially when you can follow in the footsteps of such fabulously glamorous women as Grace Kelly.

To whet your appetite, watch evocative 1956 footage of Grace entering Monte Carlo by boat in anticipation of her wedding to Prince Rainier. She wears the most divine white organdie hat! (britishpathe.com/record.php?id=59656). Follow up by seeing her rove around the French Riviera in *To Catch a Thief* (1955).

You don't have to be up for losing your house on the spin of a roulette wheel to love Monte Carlo, but it's fun to mix with the high-rolling tax exiles

FOR ARMCHAIR TRAVELLERS

WATCH *Affair in Monte Carlo* (1953): A lavish melodrama filmed on location in Monte Carlo, with Merle Oberon as a woman of substance who tries to reform compulsive gambler Richard Todd.

READ *Loser Takes All* by Graham Greene (1955): Accountant Bertram takes on the casino while on his honeymoon with spectacular results.

Monte Carlo is a city of luxury, breath-taking vistas and high stakes gambling, and the home of glamorous grown-up Grace Kelly after she married Prince Rainier of Monaco in 1956.

once in a while. Heidi Klum and Catherine Deneuve have been known to hang out in this exclusive enclave, a magnet for the discreetly rich. The **CASINO** (casino-monte-carlo.com) was designed by Charles Garnier in 1878 and is as far away from the cacophonous slot-machine gambling dens as you can get, especially if you pay a little extra to gain access to the private rooms. There, it's a veritable temple to sotto voce sophistication, as ornate and Belle Epoque as when Edward VII gambled there. Make sure you visit the **SALON BLANC**, where a mural depicts the grandes horizontales Cleo de Merode, Liane de Pougy and La Belle Otero.

If you feel the urge to gamble a bit of your hard-earned, ignore the roulette wheel in the Salle Europe – it's just too random – and head for the blackjack table in the **ENGLISH CLUB** instead. It's the only game where the odds favour the player rather than the casino, but you need to know your stuff.

The **HÔTEL DE PARIS** (montecarloresort.com) may be the costly grande dame of Monte Carlo but the upside is that being a resident allows you free access to the Spa Les Thermes Marins, the Casino and the Monte-Carlo Beach Club. Dine at the Louis XV restaurant (alain-ducasse.com) on Place du Casino. Considered to be one of the best restaurants in the world, its signature dishes include sea bass with Italian artichokes, squab pigeon with foie gras and wild strawberries with mascarpone sorbet.

'TRAVEL DOES WHAT GOOD NOVELISTS ALSO DO TO THE LIFE OF EVERYDAY, PLACING IT LIKE A PICTURE IN A FRAME OR A GEM IN ITS SETTING, SO THAT THE INTRINSIC QUALITIES ARE MADE MORE CLEAR. TRAVEL DOES THIS WITH THE VERY STUFF THAT EVERYDAY LIFE IS MADE OF, GIVING TO IT THE SHARP CONTOUR AND MEANING OF ART.'

FREYA STARK, who lived to be 100 and was the first Western woman to travel solo through the Arabian deserts.

PORTOFINO *Elizabeth Taylor Style*

FOR ARMCHAIR TRAVELLERS

READ Elizabeth von Arnim's novel, *The Enchanted April* (1922), which subtly evokes Portofino's perfumed paradise.

WATCH The movie adaptation of 1992 starring Miranda Richardson, which was filmed on location at the same wisteria-covered castle where Arnim stayed: the Castello Brown. When filming wrapped, the male lead Alfred Molina confessed to having felt a supernaturally freezing hand grasp the nape of his neck during the night-shoot and Miranda Richardson had her flapper dress yanked rather urgently by a randy Italian ghost (castellobrown.com). And you could do no worse than watch *The Barefoot Contessa* (1954), starring Ava Gardner. Many of the scenes were shot in Portofino and her couture outfits by Italian designers the Fontana sisters are beyond words!

This tiny fishing village of pretty pastel-coloured houses balanced on a rocky promontory became a jet-set hotspot in the Fifties and continues to be the summer retreat of the Italian elite. You can catch glimpses of the beautiful villa with distinctive blue shutters that belongs to the fashion designers Dolce & Gabbana nestled among the pines of Portofino, as well as Giorgio Armani's chic cream hideaway.

The post-war reconstruction and re-branding of Italy started a lifelong love for La Dolce Vita in the early 1950s and food-rationed Brits lapped up the tales of movie stars be-sporting themselves in Porto. At the centre of it all was the **HOTEL SPLENDIDO** (hotelsplendido.com), a former monastery, set in a cypress-covered hillside overlooking the Tigullio Gulf. This was the rendezvous for pairings of true international chic – the Duke and Duchess of Windsor, Rex Harrison and Lilli Palmer (before he built his 20-room, pink-washed villa, San Genosio), and Bogie and Bacall. Richard Burton and Elizabeth Taylor's romance is closely wrapped up in this town – they fled to the Splendido's Room 101 during their adulterous love affair which began on the set of the epic flop *Cleopatra* (1963).

Burton proposed to the luscious Liz over a plate of clams at **PUNY'S**, Portofino's highly chi-chi waterfront restaurant at Piazza Martiri dell'Olivetta 5. If you visit, you'll find it still has the same style food and décor, including a fab warm artichoke and octopus salad to be eaten while sitting on an original Gio Ponti chair. Mamma mia!

In 1967, Burton bought his wife an extravagant present, the motor yacht Kalizma, and she spared no expense on its $2 million refit. She filled her new sea-going love sanctuary with paintings by Degas, Monet and Van Gogh. Kalizma became a refuge from the incessant media coverage of the couple's drunken antics when moored in Portofino's pretty harbour. Liz also splashed the cash at the local designer boutiques (known as Bond Street Sur-Le-Med) and poor old Dick described her as: 'shopping like a lunatic. Elizabeth has bought umpty-nine watches, sweaters and Puccis.'

———————★———————

While schmoozing at the Hotel Splendido, cast an eye over the black-and-white photos of the hotel's most fabulous guests and sip a Prosecco cocktail or two in the Piano Bar. Brad, Angelina and George Clooney have all been spotted there. Your glass can be filled with several types (hic-hic hooray!) including the strawberry Rossini, the tangerine Puccini, raspberry Canaletto and my favourite, the gooseberry Tintoretto.

At the time of writing, a two-night stay at Hotel Splendido starts from around £1,000 per person (eek!) including breakfast and one à la carte meal (lunch or dinner). Bookings can be made through Orient-Express (orient-express.com). If that's too much, try the **SPLENDIDO MARE** (hotelsplendido. com). It's not only cheaper, but more casual – just ask Monica Bellucci, who is said to prefer it. You're also allowed to use the sister hotel's facilities.

MADRID *Ava Gardner Style*

In 1960, Ava Gardner moved to Madrid at the age of 38 to continue her lifelong love affair with Spain which started when she filmed *Pandora and the Flying Dutchman*, a high camp Surrealist fantasy in which she co-starred with James Mason in 1951. Her new home was a well-appointed apartment at 11 Avenida Doctor Arce in the chic embassy area. Directly beneath her lived the exiled President of Argentina and husband of Eva, Juan Perón. Ever the vixen, Ava used to water her carnations whenever she heard him step out onto his terrace. Her joke was to ensure the pots overflowed and cascaded below, then to scold loudly, '*Quit pissing! Spot, you terrible dog! Quit pissing on the flowers!*'

Madrid was the perfect city for Ava's vampiric tendencies as she slept by day and caroused by night, drinking at the **HOTEL RITZ** (ritzmadrid.com) until she was eventually barred for relieving herself in the lobby. She danced flamenco till dawn with gangs of gypsies, standing on tables and twirling her skirts to reveal that she was wearing no underwear and then disappearing with them for days on end.

To experience Madrid Ava-style, there's only one place to eat with the correct amount of diva-style glamour – **HORCHER** (restaurantehorcher.com). The décor is very traditional – lots

Ava Gardner struts her stuff at the Villa Rosa flamenco bar in Madrid. Mesmerized by Spanish culture, Gardner learned this Andalusian dance and even tried her hand at bull-fighting.

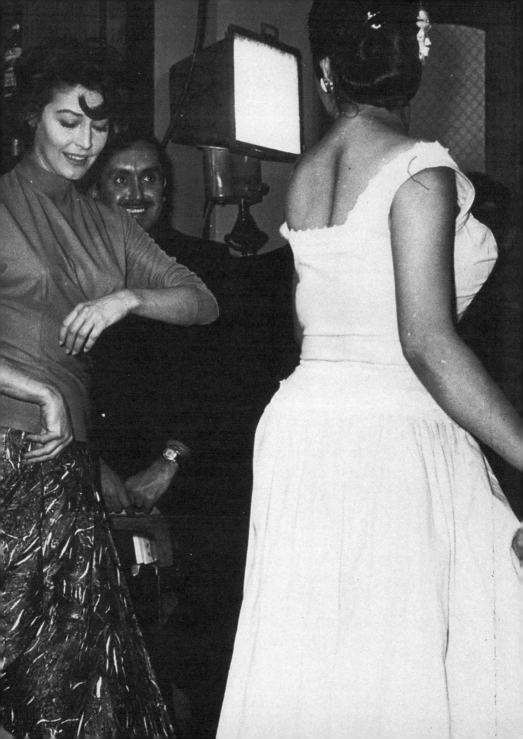

of brocade, gilt mirrors and stiff linen tablecloths. Grown-up girls be warned: discreetly hovering waiters will slip off your shoes and place your feet on plump cushions while you eat – for first-timers, this can be a little alarming! It's classic European cuisine so expect smoked salmon and blinis, lots of game including partridge, venison and roast pigeon in port wine plus a superb sea bass in saffron sauce. For dessert, try their renowned apple strudel. Ava loved it, but was banned after rather loudly voicing her complaints over the 'cheap Spanish gin' in her martini and emphasized the point by pouring her cocktail down the owner's trousers!

Another Ava haunt is still there – the **MUSEO CHICOTE** cocktail bar on Gran Via 12 (open from 8pm till 3am). Its mainly Thirties interior also features fifties chrome chairs and whiskey sours, attracting many émigré film stars including Rita Hayworth, Sophia Loren and Grace Kelly. But the one place you must visit, if you are on the Ava trail, is the **VILLA ROSA** flamenco bar, the oldest nightclub in Madrid (Plaza de Santa Ana 15).

In the 1920s Ernest Hemingway came to mingle with the picadors and listen to Manuel Morao play Spanish guitar. Writer Reid Buckley accompanied Ava in the early sixties and describes a typical soirée: 'After supper, Ava invited us out to the Villa Rosa. Waiters brought in Jamón Serrano, chorizo, salchichon and chunks of goat's cheese. The guitarist began strumming and La Paquera cleared her husky throat, humming along. Two dancers began rapping their palms in sharp, hard rhythms.' For night owls like Ava, it's open from 8pm to 6am on Saturdays!

Stay at the **INTERCONTINENTAL** (Paseo de la Castellana 49), where Ava Gardner and Frank Sinatra used to meet after their divorce for nights of love and fighting. Ava spotted Bette Davis in reception and promptly introduced herself: 'Miss Davis, I'm Ava Gardner and I'm a great fan of yours.' 'Of course you are, my dear,' said Bette. 'Of course you are.' And kept on walking.

If you want to know more about the ravishing Ava, visit the **AVA GARDNER MUSEUM** in her American birthplace at 325 E. Market St., Smithfield, NC 27577 (avagardner.org).

FOR ARMCHAIR TRAVELLERS

WATCH Pedro Almodóvar's *Broken Embraces* (2009), starring the lush Penélope Cruz and filmed in Madrid – but most films by this director will do! His *High Heels* (1991) has a sequence shot in the Villa Rosa and the opening scenes of *Tie Me Up! Tie Me Down!* (1990) were set in the Intercontinental.

READ *What's the Girl Worth?* (2003): Christina Fitzpatrick's first novel charts the first trip taken to Madrid by Catherine Kelly, a young cocktail waitress who slowly acclimatizes to life in a very different sun-drenched culture.

ST TROPEZ *Brigitte Bardot Style*

'*No road crosses St Tropez,*' wrote the rebellious novelist Colette five decades ago. 'Only one takes you there, and it doesn't go far. If you want to leave, you have to retrace your footsteps. But would you like to leave?' Well, you won't once you've visited because this Riviera honey pot is truly for the lotus-eaters among us. It's filled with playboy billionaires parking their superyachts complete with helipads in le Vieux Port and jet-setting Eurotrash tripping round the boutiques in 24-carat belly chains – a far cry from the little fishing village where Brigitte Bardot first set her kitten heels in the Fifties. After her screen debut in *And God Created Woman* (1957), the sun-tanned sexpot settled in St Tropez and is still to be found in her ten-room beachfront house.

In the Sixties St Tropez was the epicentre of a French-style sexual revolution as topless bathing hit Pamplona Beach in '64 and Bardot introduced a string of lovers, including the delectable crooner Sacha Distel, to its charms. Unless you like a crush, try to visit off-season – up to 100,000 visitors a day appear at the height of summer. Out of season, the cobbled lanes in the old fishing quarter of La Ponche are especially cute and the beaches are practically deserted.

The central square is the Place de Lices, the perfect destination for a coffee or pastis apéritif on the pavement terrace of a cool café such as **LE CAFÉ**. Don't confuse it with a newer version on the corner of the square because this was the scene of Bardot's infamous cake fights with Gunter Sachs, playboy heir to the Opel car empire, which featured the Mediterranean speciality tarte tropézienne – two slabs of sponge sandwiched together with cream.

Staying at the gorgeous **LE BYBLOS** on the Avenue Signac (byblos.com) is a must. Bardot was a frequent guest and honeymooned there with Sachs. It's built in the style of a Provençal village. Guests at Le Byblos automatically gain entry to the St Trop hot-spot Les Caves du Roy. The bar tabs are fearsome – even a glass of water can set you back an incredible sum – but while peering round its Corinthian columns you might catch sight of silver fox George Clooney.

Sit in a huge club chair and enjoy Mediterranean food with a global twist in an enchanted garden. Lanterns are hung in trees in the inside-outside space of the restaurant **SPOON** – another Alain Ducasse establishment.

If you can't get in at Byblos, a Bardot alternative is **LA PONCHE** at 3 rue des Remparts (laponche. com). Ask for a room with a terrace so that you can look out on the beach where Bardot frolicked in the waves for *And God Created Woman*.

FOR ARMCHAIR TRAVELLERS

WATCH Naturally, *And God Created Woman* (1956), directed by Bardot's ex, Roger Vadim. Our heroine jumps in and out of the beds of two brothers while writhing provocatively in her bikini.

READ Françoise Sagan's *Bonjour Tristesse* (1954), a ground-breaking novel by an 18-year-old author that introduced the world to the soigné sex of the South of France. Or for ferocious camp, try *The Hairdressers of St Tropez* (1995) by Madonna's best mate, the naughty Rupert Everett.

GROWN-UP GLAMOUR *Travel Tips*

★ *'To lose your prejudices, you must travel.'*
MARLENE DIETRICH

★ Take care with your passport photo – you'll have to look at that unfortunate cast to your eye for the next ten years if you don't! After a long flight, you don't want to see immigration officials from Minsk to the Maldives stifling grins as they let you through. Wear something white to direct the light onto your face and get rid of any double chins by slightly jutting your chin straightforward like a turtle emerging from its shell. It works, promise!

★ Before you pack your suitcase lay all your clothes out and count your money. Now halve the amount of clothes and double the cash and you'll be about right!

★ I'm of the same opinion as Orson Welles, who once said: 'There are only two emotions in a plane: boredom and terror.' There's also the risk of deep vein thrombosis (DVT) on long-haul flights, so my trick is to ask for an aisle seat. This means that you'll be forced to get up regularly when your seatmates need to get something out of the overhead lockers, visit the bathroom, et al.

★ **BRITT EKLAND** says, 'I aim for five hours' sleep on a twelve-hour flight so that I don't feel wrecked at the other end. Then when everyone is tucking into the crummy breakfast, I go in and hog the bathroom. I take my entire kit and wash my face, hands, underarms and any other place that needs freshening up, and come back totally refreshed, with teeth brushed.'

★ **LISA KUDROW** buys thick paper napkins, soaks them in almond oil and then puts them in individual plastic bags. Whenever she's travelling, she uses them to refresh and moisturize her skin.

★ *'As the traveller who has once been from home is wiser than he who has never left his own doorstep, so a knowledge of one other culture should sharpen our ability to scrutinize more steadily, to appreciate more lovingly, our own.'* **MARGARET MEAD**, the most significant anthropologist of the twentieth century, who was still having new books published at the age of 74.

★ Finally, the greatest tip of all comes from **ERNEST HEMINGWAY**: *'Never go on trips with anyone you do not love.'* Enough said!

8

AFFAIRS *of the Heart*

Glamorous grown-ups redefine what it is to be older; the traditional rules about love and marriage no longer apply. In the past, the driving force in many a relationship was economic security – at some point a woman would spend time at home looking after her offspring while the man took full responsibility for financing the domestic sphere. Not so today, when many women have achieved our own success and don't need to rely on the contents of a man's wallet.

Some of us, like Sharon Stone and Cameron Diaz, are single and happy; others are merrily ensconced with a partner and family just like Catherine Zeta-Jones and Jennifer Lopez; some of us are single parents through choice or force of circumstance and bringing up children on our own like Teri Hatcher; many of us have chosen not to have kids at all like Kim Cattrall and a few of us are staying at home and looking after their man in the traditional way. But the most important thing to remember as we navigate the ups and downs of our romantic lives is that, as twenty-first-century women, we have the right to choose.

Cary Grant and Ingrid Bergman in Hitchcock's *Notorious* (1946) features one of the most famous screen kisses in movie history clocking in at a little over three minutes.

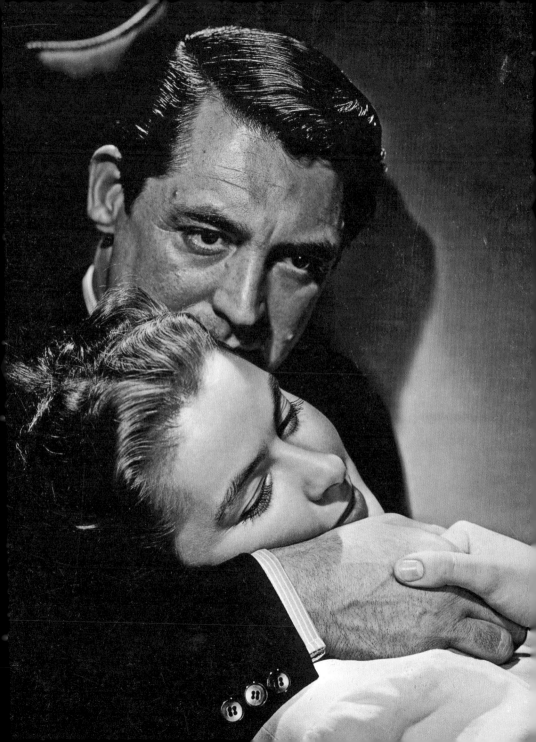

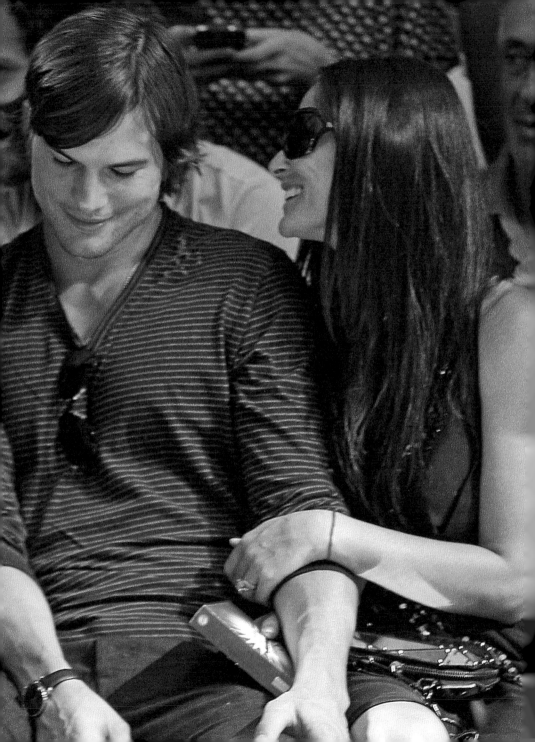

THE MYTH *of the Cougar*

In the last couple of years the 'cougar' has entered into the lexicon of words used to describe the older woman, especially in relation to affairs of the heart. Cougars are, according to the media image, a new race of predatory female: all Botoxed-up and miniskirted, prowling the urban jungle in search of their prey. Of course, this is a double-edged term: some see it as empowering – if fifty-something men can run off with teenage blondes, why can't women do the same with a series of nubile toy-boys? At the same time, it seems slightly contradictory: if we think that the men who do it are suffering a midlife crisis and look more than a little daft, why should a woman get away with it? Trading a spouse in purely for a younger model is cruel, whatever your sex.

As Michelle Obama says: 'Cute's good. But cute only lasts for so long, and then it's "Who are you as a person?" Don't look at the bankbook or the title. Look at the heart. Look at the soul. When you're dating a man, you should always feel good … You shouldn't be in a relationship with somebody who doesn't make you completely happy and make you feel whole.' Drew Barrymore puts it even more simply: 'I think women just want a guy who's going to be on the level with them and chivalrous and sweet and a good partner.'

When Demi Moore met Ashton Kutcher in 2003 she called it a 'life-changing evening. I knew it had the potential to be something special right away.' When they married in 2005 the bride was 42 and the groom 27.

Glamorous grown-ups such as Demi Moore, whose husband Ashton Kutcher is 15 years younger than her, or a 40-plus Mariah Carey, 11 years older and a few squillion richer than her partner Nick Cannon, are held up as perfect examples of the cougar trend – although in Demi's case, in particular, it seems to devalue what appears to be a highly successful partnership that works because of who they are. She recognizes that she's been '…plucked out as a bit of a poster girl. I don't know why that is, but I just kind of step back and sometimes say, "There is a reason, and what is it that I have to say in a positive way?"' Glamorous grown-up Courtney Cox, whose sitcom *Cougar Town* has done much to familiarize us with the term, says: 'I used to think a cougar was a woman who had lots of plastic surgery, who was trying to look younger, and dating what she thought was her contemporary even though she was so much older. Now I just think it's a woman who's confident, who uses her experience and her confidence to date younger guys. There are a lot of men who actually are more attracted to older women because there's no game-playing.'

★

If, as a potential cougar, you're wondering how low you can go, this is the grown-up girls' golden rule: half your age plus seven, so if you're 40, it's 27, while fifties can date a man of 32, and so on. (That's why Madonna, 50+, and model squeeze Jesus, just in his twenties, feels a little icky!)

THE *Ideal* MAN

SOPHIA LOREN says: 'I have often thought of an ideal man, created him in my mind's eye, and, in my opinion, he is a failure. In the first place he would be faultless, and what could be more monotonous than a man who does not provoke some healthy negative reaction? Who could live with a man who is so perfectly handsome, charming and imbued with the character of a saint? If your eyes are completely clouded with a vision that you have made up from movie stars and other famous men, a vision that bears little resemblance to the man before you, you are bound to be disappointed.

'Once we have past the dreamy stage of adolescence we have no need for such a man. For a handsome face and a graceful figure will not satisfy a mature woman. She is ready for the real challenge of love that admits imperfection and ambiguity. So what I have to say to you about love is not about film stars, it is about the man or men in your life – the one across the breakfast table or the one you're waiting to meet. That man, because he's right for you in some strange and unpredictable way, is not less than ideal, he is your ideal.'

HAPPY EVER AFTER:
Iman and Bowie

This glamorous power couple met on a blind date at a friend's dinner party and a year later, rock god David proposed to supermodel Iman on a boat trip in Paris. Married in 1992, they plighted their troth with his 'n' hers tattoos. Now they've been together for more than 20 years, with a child each from former marriages and one together after years of IVF. Iman says of their relationship: 'David and I had done it all separately and then we found each other. I still fancy him and he makes me laugh like no one else does. Sometimes it feels like we've been married for forty years, and sometimes it's like we just met, but I really feel as if I've known him all my life. When you're young you think of love in terms of fireworks, but I think women need more emotional security, and he is there for me all the time, which is something which has never happened to me before.' As for David… '*You'd think that a rock star being married to a supermodel would be the best thing in the world – it is.*'

DATING *Après Divorce*

Not all of us are as lucky as Mr and Mrs Bowie and sometimes things don't work out the way they should. If you're feeling a little downcast after divorce, take heed of Phoebe from *Friends*, who says, quite rightly: 'It's time to get out of the bitter barn and play in the hay!' So if your husband has run off with the bunny that he met at the gym (twenty years younger than you, toned, oiled and tango-tanned); if your boyfriend has left you for a hairy man or if you've never experienced the pleasures of the flesh at all, you may be asking yourself fundamental questions such as, 'What am I doing wrong?' Whatever the reason for your single state, as Courtney Cox tells her best buddy Jennifer Aniston, 'You've just got to be willing to put yourself out there, there are people in the same situation. You're not alone.'

First dates après divorce can so easily turn into the last rites because, although we are constantly told that there are wonderful men out there, many of them quite patently are not. You're bound to encounter some oddities on the road to romantic happiness, but if you want a charming beau to sweep you off your feet, you must learn to laugh in the face of adversity while pressing on to the next assignation. As Mae West advised: '*Don't cry for a man who's left you, the next one may fall for your smile.*'

WHERE TO FIND A MAN
(If You Really Want One)

Men are like stars, they come out at night and there are a couple of traditional habitats in which they are sure to be spotted. The first is the sports bar – an airless enclave, pungent with testosterone, where men gaze at jumbo screens, their only sound a slurred whooping when a guy scores a goal while simultaneously gelling his hair. There is also the latest 'hot' club in which scantily clad teenagers and leering Lotharios act out bizarre mating rituals involving huge quantities of cocaine and donor kebabs. Obviously these are not the places for a glamorous grown-up like you.

SCENE ONE: A SINGLES NIGHT

Singles nights can be fun. Really. At least everyone's there for the same reason, although strangely, the same sort of beauty hierarchy exists there as anywhere. The notion that judgments should be made on good looks rather than personality still apply and singles nights remain a microcosm of the real, cruel world. If a man is good-looking, he will be mobbed.

As you stare into this maw of death, try bluffing confidence: the more you fake it, the more you feel it. Here are some other survival tactics:

★ Go with a friend – at least you can have a giggle together.

★ If it's an evening event in a bar, enter with style: head up and shoulders back with a smile on your face rather than tottering in like a shot dog.

★ ★ ★ ★ ★ ★ ★ ★ ★ ★ ★ ★

★ The more you pay to attend a singles night, the more the pool of dates will improve and they'll probably be more serious about it. Most cities have a thriving singles scene and it's really easy to find reviews and figure out the best operators by searching on the internet.

★ Don't go to anything that involves dancing. They do it differently these days and it usually involves rubbing up against another woman.

————★————

Going it alone? Give yourself a break and pick an event that has some sort of content such as a gallery visit, a wine tasting or a singles book club. You don't have to go in cold to a conversation and events will happen naturally around you.

SCENE TWO: PERSONAL ADS

There's a stigma attached to personal ads and lonely hearts' columns. We may feel that the correct way to click is by falling into animated conversation across a Brazilian beach bar or at a Gregorian chant recital; you might be waiting for the runes to foretell the moment your soul-mate's path will cross yours and believe that fate and karma hold the key, but life's not like that. We're (mostly) all too rushed to follow through that sidelong glance on the escalator, so personal ads are a practical way of getting singles together and cutting out the married/attached/gay. There are many publications within which to place your personal ad. Obviously if you go for the free ads, you'll be inundated with responses from sharp-suited men in search of a green card. Here are some ideas to get you started:

★ Choose the paper whose target audience best matches your own profile. So if you love fox hunting, regard any heir to the throne as delicious and think that Belville Sassoon taffeta evening gowns worn with a black velvet Alice band are the last word in sophistication, then the *Daily Telegraph* is for you. *The Daily Mail* is for anyone who hates single mothers or asylum seekers and *Loot* is for losers. *Guardian* Soulmates is one of the best and it has an easy-to-work website too.

★ If the ad has a voicemail, listen carefully. You can learn a lot from a man's intonation and if you instinctively recoil from his honeyed tones, *DO NOT DATE HIM!*

SCENE THREE: INTERNET SITES

Be wary of these: often the most popular appear to have been co-opted by predatory polygamists or Columbian money-launderers. What's more, you can get a completely false impression of somebody from a blurred photo and the gift of the gab.

★

damedating.com reviews all the dating websites for ease of use, the quality of dates and the people who have signed up to them, plus their experiences. Some of the big sites come out really badly – you have been warned!

★ The best sites are the less corporate ones and include mysinglefriend.com. If you're looking for a bearded intellectual, try ivorytowers.net.

SCENE FOUR: THE SHOW AND TELL PARTY

Spread the word to your girlfriends that you're holding a party but they can only come if they bring a single man. The men will already have been vetted, you can get all the goss on them, everyone is automatically introduced and the more people you invite, the more men there will be. All the glamorous singles will love you!

MEN *What Not To Date*

1 Don't go out with men who live in rented accommodation.

2 Don't date men who have to go home early to bathe their parents.

3 Avoid men with criminal records (I'm thinking Madonna's 'American Pie' here).

4 Also men who advertise for friends in free magazines.

5 Remember, a date full of ambiguities and tension will inevitably lead to a relationship full of ambiguities and tension.

6 And any man who says '*You're too good for me*' is probably right!

FIRST DATE *Fashion*

It's a minefield! Now you've bagged a date with a delicious man – what do you wear? What worries a lot of us is the visual information that you're immediately putting out to a potential partner. Make sure he gets the right message with the following tips:

★ Don't put everything in the shop window – unless all you're after is a quick bunk-up after closing time. The obvious rule is that if you want to show a hint of cleavage, keep your legs covered up (and vice versa).

★ By all means, flash a cute pair of pins but only in black opaque tights and avoid any that have shine in them – they always make legs look like over-processed sausages. Despite Anna Wintour going out with bare legs in the depths of a New York winter, it can look a bit vulgar on a first date. (And remember, Wintour's bare legs speak volumes: she's telling you that she only needs to totter a few yards from the front row seat of a Galliano show to her chauffeur-driven limo to her huge hotel suite. The rest of us must make do with public transport.)

★ Don't overdress to make a good impression and unless you want to come across as a femme fatale, avoid piling on the make-up.

★ Do dress smartly enough to show him that you've made an effort.

★ Leave the red lipstick and leopard print at home until you feel you know him better. Glamorous grown-up Katherine Heigl does it this way round: *'I find a sexy outfit OK on the first date – even on the second and third. But if you've the fourth date and it's still only about appearance and being a sex-bomb, something must be wrong.'*

★ Don't wear a new outfit because you'll feel uncomfortable.

★ No leather trousers or 'witty' hats.

★ You can't go wrong with an LBD, mid-heel slingback pumps and a pastel pashmina/shrug/wrap. Charm bracelet and chignon are practically obligatory.

'I PREFER OLDER WOMEN – THEY HAVE SEEN MORE, HEARD MORE, AND KNOW MORE THAN A DEMURE YOUNG GIRL. I'LL TAKE AN OLDER WOMAN EVERY TIME. '

CLARK GABLE

SIX *Who Scored On Set*

1 KATHARINE HEPBURN and Spencer Tracy: *Woman of the Year* (1942)

2 LAUREN BACALL and Humphrey Bogart: *To Have and Have Not* (1944)

3 INGRID BERGMAN and director Roberto Rossellini: *Stromboli* (1950)

4 ELIZABETH TAYLOR and Richard Burton: *Cleopatra* (1961)

5 GOLDIE HAWN and Kurt Russell: *Swing Shift* (1983)

6 SUSAN SARANDON and Tim Robbins: *Bull Durham* (1988)

GIVING *the Right Impression*

Assuming it's all going well and you've invited him back to yours, here are a few tips on making the right kind of impression.

★ Hide any 'Best of' CDs – often men will attach importance to your choice of music as it tells them something about you. It's a bit cheesy, say, to have the Top Ten Operatic Arias on one disk instead of each opera in full. Another trap to avoid is obvious power pop compilations along the lines of That's What I Call Music No. 152, or Music to Drive By. It's perfectly fine to allow a prospective mate a peep through the window of your forbidden pleasures, though – such as your crush on Neil Diamond or David Essex. It will loosen him up and who knows, he may reveal a few naughty secrets of his own! But MC Hammer or Daniel O'Donnell will never be cool.

★ It might be tempting to pick out the latest literary work and prop it up, cover forward, on the bookshelf, but this will look like a desperate display of your intellectual credentials. By all means give him a glimpse of your personality, but royal biographies are most definitely out, as are triumph-over-tragedy tomes such as *I Was Born in a Tipperary Slum* or *Sweet Jesus, Stop the Pain*. For your own sanity, if not his, bin them at once!

★ Keep all pets out of bounds: you don't want an unexpected threesome with your pedigree Bedlington Terrier.

★ Remove all family photos – the focus should be on you, not your talented offspring or collection of exes, no matter how searing their good looks or heart-thumping their celebrity credibility. And any photo of your mother is taboo, too – her sinister bi-focal gaze will follow him round the room like a baleful version of the *Mona Lisa*.

★ Prune your DVDs and especially be sure to remove anything starring Jennifer Aniston. She's one of those heroines that women love (she's one of us!) but men find strangely neurotic. Never display your Pilates collection either – he should think that hot bod is the result of genetics, but if you happen to have a taste for Spaghetti Westerns... Bingo! Flash-forward to a cinematic clinch to the haunting strains of Ennio Morricone.

★ Men hate ornaments! They think they are pointless dust-collectors and the worst sight to confront them is a collection of ceramic frogs, pigs or commemorative teaspoons. Naturally, your exquisite taste should already preclude this calamity!

THOUGHTS *on First-Date Kisses*

'If you kiss on the first date and it's not right, then there will be no second date. Sometimes it's better to hold out and not kiss for a long time. I am a strong believer in kissing being very intimate, and the minute you kiss, the floodgates open for everything else.'
JENNIFER LOPEZ

'A kiss can be a comma, a question mark or an exclamation point. That's basic spelling that every woman ought to know.'
MISTINGUETT

'A kiss is a lovely trick designed by nature to stop speech when words become superfluous.'
INGRID BERGMAN

'I prefer a kiss that is so much more than just a tongue in your mouth.'
KATHERINE HEIGL

'He is a supersexy, hot kisser and he is sexy to me because he can be singing in front of 25,000 people one minute and the next be changing our daughter's diaper.'
HEIDI KLUM ON SEAL

In 2004 Seal proposed to Heidi Klum on top of a 14,000 ft high glacier in the Canadian Rockies. She says, 'He had an igloo built there, rose petals everywhere, candles. No trees, nothing – it was hardcore. I was ecstatic.'

'Too much make-up has ruined many a kiss.'
MAE WEST

'A guy can just as easily dump you if you fuck him on the first date as he can if you wait until the tenth.'
KIM CATTRALL

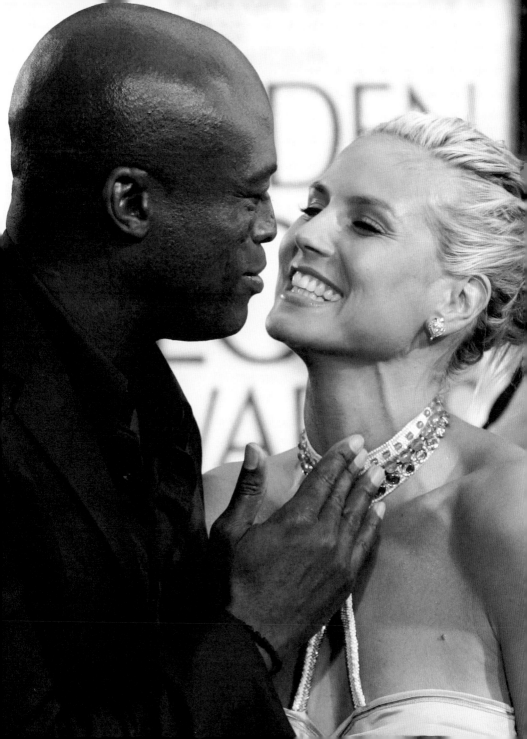

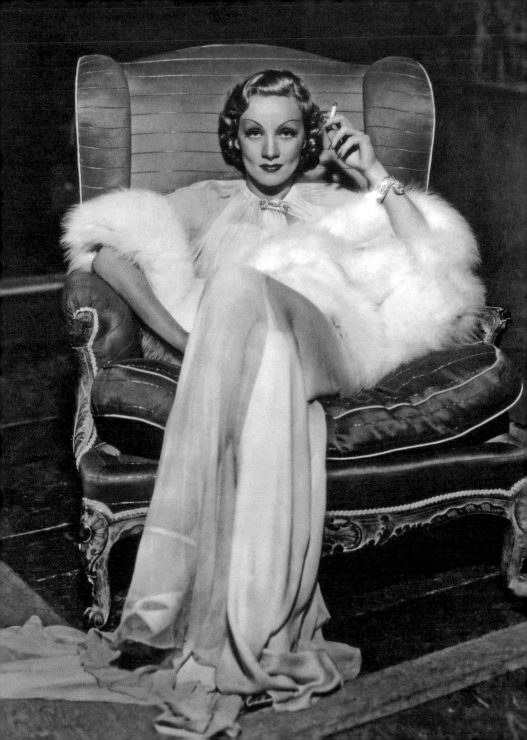

DRESSING FOR A DATE
by Marlene Dietrich

'When you have a dinner date, be prepared so that you can dress without delay. Be ready on time. Even if you should appear a dream personified, and he has waited hours to take the dream to dinner, you've spoiled the evening. His over-hungry stomach won't let his eyes see all your beauty, his mood is bad, and by the time he's had his coffee and his mood is fine, you are quite angry and not beautiful.'

Marlene Dietrich vamps it up with the legendary legs that were the opening close-up of the film *Desire* (1926). She said, 'Darling, the legs aren't so beautiful, I just know what to do with them.'

HOW TO *Keep the Spark Alive*

Whatever the length of your relationship, it's always good to put in a bit of time and effort to keep things electric between you. Set the scene for an intimate evening by creating the right mood with soft shadows, sweet music and scented candles. If you haven't already, install a dimmer switch or buy some additional low-level lamps – you can transform the whole ambience of a room with just the simple flick of a switch.

★ If a classic seduction is your goal, furnishings and fabrics should be subtly tactile: velvet, chenille and suede cushions will soften the hard lines of a leather sofa. Moving on to the bedroom, who could fail to be stirred by a set of crisp Egyptian cotton sheets with a shot-silk throw?

HEAVEN SCENT: THE BEST LUXURY CANDLES

★ **DIPTYQUE** (diptyqueparis.com) is quite simply the world leader in a crowded market. Founded in 1961, this French company uses only natural ingredients and the fifty-plus fragrances range from simple to heady and complex. In my experience most men love 'L'Eau', one of the original scents and based on a sixteenth-century recipe for potpourri and composed of a clove pomander with notes of cinnamon, geranium, sandalwood and rose. Jennifer Lopez has Diptyque on her rider.

★ **TOCCA** (tocca.com) are more minimalist in their presentation and therefore well suited to modernist interiors. The 'Havana' and 'Blood Orange' are gorge fragrances, while Grace is fantastic for summer romance when you don't want anything too cloying.

★ **VOTIVO** candles (votivo.com) are hand-poured in the USA using the finest soy wax and purvey the most maverick of aromas to grown-up girl Madonna, including 'Rain', 'White Ocean Sands', 'Prairie Sage' and 'Tuscan Olive'. Note: This label is often featured in men's magazines and is reckoned to be a bit rock star!

★ **JO MALONE** candles (jomalone.co.uk) are among the most expensive but as with any fragrance, you get what you pay for. The cost of a three-combination, four-wick whopper is somewhat staggering, though! 'Pomegranate Noir' is the most seductive of her scents, originally inspired by the look and feel of a red silk dress. Notes of pomegranate, raspberry, plum and pink pepper combine with patchouli, frankincense and spicy woods to create the most evocative of aromas.

GOING *Undercover*

Married, monogamous or on the prowl, glamorous grown-ups have been skilled in the art of seduction for much of our history. Think Madame Du Barry reclining on a buttercup silk chaise longue with her white greyhound Mirza resplendent in a diamond collar, or Anne Bancroft as Mrs Robinson rolling down black seamed stockings in *The Graduate* (1967), for erotic *mise en scène* conjured out of midnight black lace and intoxicating perfume.

Many of us today don't realize our own potent force, a quality that can render grown men weak. There's a tendency to focus on our irregularities – the bits that show the tracks of time or the vicissitudes of childbirth. OK, you might be a little less taut but that shouldn't deter you from a night of passion – besides, you have the most seductive of offensive weapons to wield: luxurious lingerie. Anyway, if love really is blind, how come suspenders are so popular?

Lingerie is the ultimate artifice and can be used to create an incredible expectation of delight in our partners. It's far sexier to flash a glimpse of stocking – any wrapped object is more mysterious and compelling than one that stands there starkly unadorned, that's why blush-pink tissue paper was invented! Think of your body as the best kind of Christmas present, something delicious just waiting to be unwrapped.

'STOCKINGS NEVER FAIL TO MAKE YOU FEEL SEXY. I LIKE HOLD-UPS, BUT THE PROBLEM IS IF YOU'VE GOT TOO MUCH MEAT AT THE TOP, YOU GET A BULGE THERE. SO I OFTEN WEAR THOSE OVER-THE-KNEE FRENCH SCHOOLGIRL SOCKS. '

NIGELLA LAWSON

WHAT LIES *Beneath*

THE BRASSIÈRE

As the years go by and breast-feeding plus gravity take their toll on our pups, most of us need more support. The first step is to be measured properly. Rigby and Peller (rigbyandpeller.com) have been bestriding the market as the Colossus of underwear since 1939 and offer an expert fitting and bespoke service. The right fit is much more comfortable; also thrillingly transformative: by hoisting your embonpoint up into the right position, you'll create a waist and lose 20 pounds (without cutting back on white chocolate) in the process. What's more, any type of breast – from pancake to spaniel's ears – can be transformed into a knock 'em dead décolleté.

Despite what the middle market tells you, you will get a better-quality bra if you pay more. Look for a bra that combines the right combination of support and erotic allure. Wacoal (wacoal.com) and Le Mystère (lemystere.com) are perfect for sexy standard and voluptuous plus sizes.

BRIEF ENCOUNTERS

Rounded tummies and plump thighs can be disguised with a chemise and French knickers or a teddy (camisole and knickers in one). If you are a little shy, remember that a teddy slips from the shoulders and has to be taken off before the fun can begin – for many of us, too much over-exposure on the first night with a new partner can be slightly scary, so why not opt for an Empire-line peignoir or embroidered kimono instead? Labels such as La Perla, Cosabella, Chantal Thomass and Myla are more costly but high quality. Like a Rolls-Royce they're built to last, so why not indulge? For panties, think Lejaby (lejaby.com), a Lyon label that has many styles with full-rear coverage – always a plus! Here are some more ideas for you to think about:

★ Corsets and bustiers can give a waist and push up the breasts – and you don't have to remove them before getting down and dirty.

★ French knickers or boy shorts look much better than a thong at any age. Try Betsey Johnson Intimates (betseyjohnson. com) for a range of styles and sizes plus a dose of good old-school glamour.

★ Aussie beauty Elle Macpherson (ellemacphersonintimates. com) believes matching lingerie is 'absolutely essential – it just makes you feel better. I mean, you wouldn't walk around with one blue sock and one red sock would you? If I'm wearing a bra that doesn't match the knickers, I feel like I'm walking with a limp – it just doesn't feel right.'

★ Bette Davis once revealed: '*I often think that a slightly exposed shoulder emerging from a long satin nightgown packs more sex than two naked bodies in bed.*'

★ High heels are perfect for bedtime. They lengthen the legs for starters and you can keep the really high Louboutin mules for the bedroom – believe me, you won't be walking in them!

STRIP *and Tease*

What better way to show off your lingerie to your other half than by doing a saucy strip? To keep things suitably glamorous, take your cue from burlesque – it's easier to be camp sexy rather than raunchy sexy and one of the benefits of learning the art of the Fifties strip is that you appear to reveal all without actually doing so. Enhancing the charms while revealing little only heightens sexual imagination.

1 Choose an outfit with sex appeal rather than one that is tired and familiar – grey sweats and Uggs won't set the right mood. Err on the side of elegance. Never underestimate the importance of accessories such as jewellery, gloves, stockings and heels. Role play might help you get over any embarrassment. Pick a character in the driving seat, but flirtatiously so – leave policewomen and naughty matrons to those with less imagination!

2 Place a chair in the middle of the room and put on the right music. This is crucial – if you put on Britney Spears' 'Slave 4 U' you'll be setting yourself up for comparison and quite frankly, it's not fair on Britney! Ravel's 'Bolero' or 'Carmina Burana' are too frightening and you'll be the one with performance anxiety.

3 Invite him in and ask him to sit down on the sofa. Tell him the guideline is no touching! Throughout your routine, keep communicating with your eyes – it's like reaching out and touching without saying a word.

4 Now work the room, shaking what your mama gave you. Walk with one foot in front of the other as if you are on a tightrope while pausing to do a slow bump and grind – remember, it's a leisurely circular movement, not a back-and-forth thrust of the hips à la demented Doberman!

5 Start removing your clothes but take it sloooow! Long-sleeved gloves first: remove each finger, then pull off with an elegant flourish and let them flutter to the floor. Removing the jacket is a key move and this should be slowly unbuttoned while you have your back to him. Glance over your shoulder in a playful way with one eyebrow raised and then shrug so that your jacket slowly falls down your back. Remove your arms from each sleeve and then slowly turn round with the jacket clutched demurely over your breasts. Smile seductively and then let it fall.

6 Sashay to the chair and put one leg up at a time to remove your shoes and stockings. Look right in his eyes as you kick each shoe off, then roll each stocking down, point your toes as you slip them over your feet and then discard.

7 Now turn away from him and while arching your back, start to undo your skirt. Let it drop to the floor and elegantly step out. Don't let your OCD take over at this point so you start hanging things up in the closet – it will break the mood!

8 You're working up to the final reveal! Turn away from him and undo your bra. Release each arm, then turn and face him with your bra clutched against your naked breasts. Turn your back again and toss the garment over one shoulder so it hits him lightly in the face. Let sexual havoc ensue!

BURLESQUE MOVIES *to Inspire Your Moves*

★ **LADY OF BURLESQUE** *(1943)* A murder-mystery set in a burlesque theatre with the divine Barbara Stanwyck as performer Dixie Daisy.

★ **GYPSY** *(1962)* Starring Natalie Wood and Rosalind Russell, it charts the rise to fame of iconic stripper Gypsy Rose Lee.

★ **THE NIGHT THEY RAIDED MINSKY'S** *(1968)* Bombshell Britt Ekland plays an innocent Amish girl from Smoketown, Pennsylvania, who although desperate to perform her Bible dances on stage, inadvertently invents the striptease.

★ **VARIETEASE** and **TEASERAMA** *(both 1954)* Re-released double bill of burlesque performers, including Tempest Storm and the notorious Bettie Page, who performs her renowned 'Dance of the Seven Veils'.

★ **TOO HOT TO HANDLE** *(1960)* Jaded stripper Midnight Franklin, played by voluptuous Jayne Mansfield, works at the Pink Flamingo Club in London and does a variety of burlesque routines, including one in a feather-bedecked swimsuit.

Ursula Andress in *Up to His Ears* (1965), in which she performs a reverse strip by putting on, rather than taking off her clothes, behind a fan. One critic described her as 'magnificently statuesque'.

★ **BLAZE** *(1989)* Paul Newman plays a Louisiana governor who falls in love with stripper Blaze Starr. The amazing Dianne Brill has a bit part as stripper Delilah Dough, who performs her act out of a giant clamshell!

★ And last but not least: **YESTERDAY, TODAY, AND TOMORROW** *(1963)*, where Sophia Loren does a sexy routine after training with the strippers at the Crazy Horse in Paris.

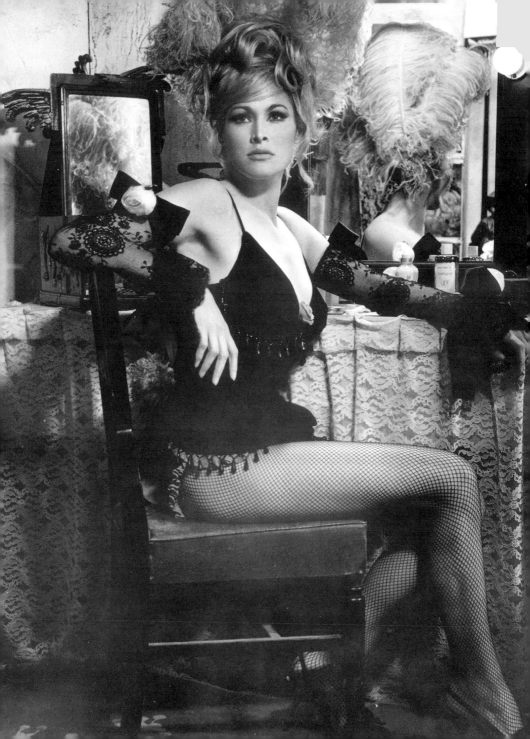

9

SURVIVAL *Instincts*

Today, women live longer than they ever have done, but cultural attitudes do not always keep up with us – it's how ageing is perceived that's often out of date, not our fabulous selves! Think of yourself as that supremely enigmatic Renaissance symbol, the mulberry tree, which flowers late in a burst of beautiful, compelling blooms. (Mulberries can also be rejuvenated with a good pruning, see chapter 5.)

Being older means being able to shed a lot of the stuff that has bothered many a grown-up girl in the past – striving for perfection, the need to please, keeping up with the latest looks. Fashion is clearly a fun indulgence, especially flipping through the pages of *Vogue Italia* and gasping at the latest Paolo Roversi photo-shoot as you sip your café au lait. But chasing after cheap copies of every fad in Zara can look a bit desperate, and when you find yourself dressing like your daughter you'd better start saving for her therapist. These days, standing out from the crowd should be less to do with having the perfect body and more about displaying your innate and exquisite taste. You can be the woman to be reckoned with!

GROWING OLDER *Means Less Responsibility*

You may not have felt the need to indulge yourself, or perhaps not had the confidence in the past. For most of us, it seems, other people – particularly our children – have always come first. Now the rug-rats can fend for themselves it's time to break out and do your own thing.

Don't feel guilty about it, either. Oscar-winning actress Tilda Swinton is refreshingly upfront about the delights of spending time apart from her twins: 'I think I enjoy my work now even more, simply because it's even easier than it was. It sounds sacrilegious to say that anything's a delight when you're away from your children, but the truth is that it is refreshing to only have yourself to dress in the morning, and to lie diagonally across the bed. Making films, going round the world on tour – all those crazy things that were so difficult before are so much easier than breastfeeding twins for 14 months, that frankly, it is a delight.'

It's time for you to look to yourself again with a benign and loving eye, to find out what you really want. It may be nothing – perhaps you are entirely happy (let's meet so you can tell me your secret!), or you may have a hankering to see the Northern Lights, or watch the sun set over the Taj Mahal (although that didn't make Princess Di any happier). At first, this newfound freedom can be frightening but now it really is up to you to choose to be happy or not. You are equally free to be a miserable old trout, but I know which life I prefer. Let's face it, growing old is something you only do if you're lucky!

AGE REALLY IS *Just A Number*

The age we fear depends on the age we are. At 16, I remember seeing 21 as inconceivably far off; at 30 most of us dread 40, and at 40 we are absolutely petrified of turning 50. But I'm here to tell you – it ain't so bad! All the fears that we have about growing older are in our own heads, created by the cultural attitudes around us. But over these anxieties, we can have mastery, domination and control!

As I see it, people can be just as old when they're numerically young, anyway. When I was at school, some of the little boys already acted as if they were little old men, and it's taken 40 years for their bodies to catch up with their minds! Conversely, I don't really believe that I've evolved too far from that 17-year-old peroxide punk with a penchant for singing along to the Buzzcocks' 'Spiral Scratch (B'dum B'dum)'. Time is a relative concept, so don't let it dominate your life – as Gloria Swanson said: *'I think all this talk about age is foolish. Every time I'm one year older, everyone else is too.'* Alternatively you could take Eva Gabor's approach: *'I believe in loyalty. When a woman reaches a certain age, she should stick with it.'*

AN INCREASE IN YOUR AGE
Means an Increase in Your Power

You know more and you have wisdom, so use it! The beautiful thing about ageing is that you have now learned to value experience, something you turned your nose up at when you were young. Experience equals confidence, which in turn gives us independence – and the result? Complete freedom just when we have the time and (hopefully) money to enjoy it! What's more, unlike the Gossip Girls out there, you are less subject to the whims and vagaries of fashion. As Meg Ryan says: 'I think 40 is a really meaningless statistic, I really do. I have had much more seminal changes, much more distinct than 40. And also, I don't think it has the same meaning as it did to our parents. What I like, and I felt this way at 38, is that I have some confidence in my experience and my ability to judge my experience. You can relax. I feel like it's become this whole process of acceptance and relaxing, and not about that stuff that happens when you're younger – about pleasing other people or second-guessing yourself – which is a huge fucking waste of time! If it's taken me this much time to get here, then I'm just grateful, whatever age I am.'

AGEING *Is Not a Disease*

Although many are trying to call it a medical condition and thus seek a cure, just because you've hit 40, 50 or 60, it doesn't mean that your life is over – it's just, well… a bit different. And there's no point in being preoccupied with your weight and wrinkles (lucky you, if that's all that bothers you), particularly if it's preventing you from doing anything else with your life. As Britt Ekland says, 'You don't have to be a movie star, a celebrity, a rich woman or born beautiful – somewhere along the line, beauty fades. You have got to be alone with yourself for a while and not preoccupied with that beautiful handbag in the shop window or tonight's dinner. You've got to look at yourself really hard. Think about what you want to achieve. Most people automatically say, "I'll start tomorrow." If you say "tomorrow", you have already failed because there is always another tomorrow. It's got to happen right this minute, your head has got to say "today"!'

Jerry Hall is confident enough to show a hint of grey roots. She says, 'I don't buy anything that says "anti-ageing". I think it's insulting and ageist.'

If you've always lived off your looks and are not as philosophical as Britt, the patina of age that your face and body begins to display may not be as appealing to you as it would be when applied to a nineteenth-century animalier bronze or the fine façade of Derbyshire's Haddon Hall. Jean Shrimpton, the most beautiful of the Sixties supermodels, found it hard saying (when 48!): 'I'm middle-aged. The body is packing up. I can't see any redeeming feature in getting older. You just think, "Nature's had you, you're on the scrap heap."'

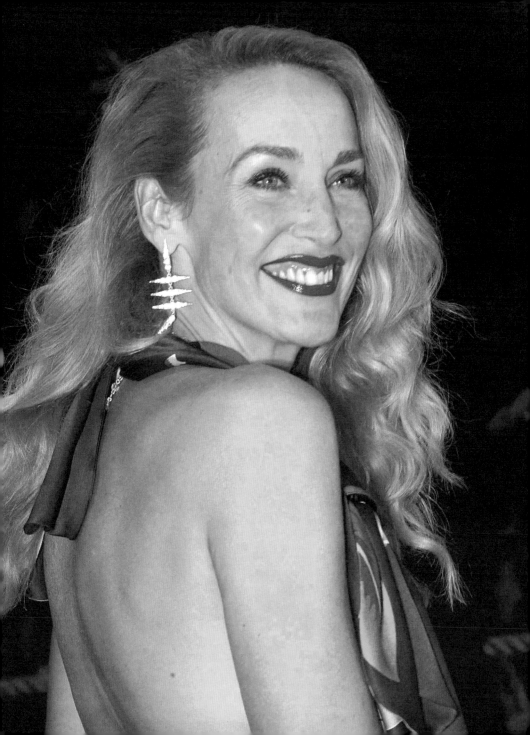

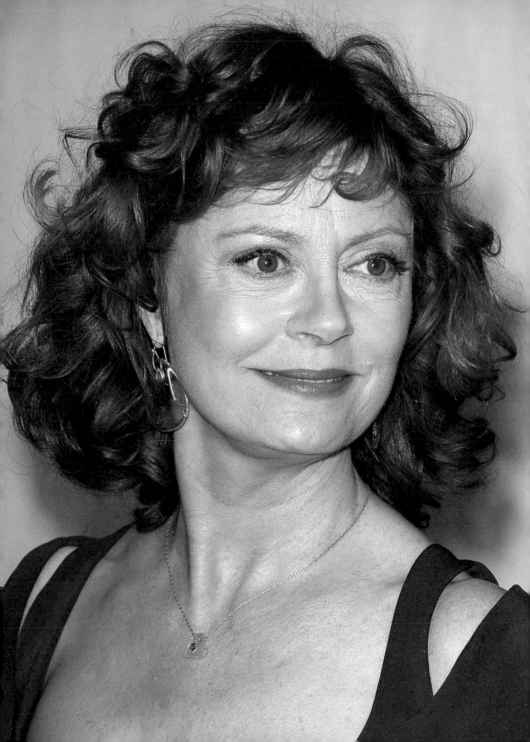

Maybe Jean has a rather melancholic personality, but my reality is a little different. Focusing on how you look today compared to how you looked ten years ago is self-defeating, even self-absorbing. In doing so, you are turning inward instead of outward, so turn around and unfurl your petals to the sun (but give yourself a break and do this while slathered in the best sunscreen). Susan Sarandon advises: *'Anything that makes you feel passionate and makes you laugh helps you to stay young. When you are engaged in the bigger picture, you can't afford the space to become so self-involved that everything is a crisis for you. Grassroots activism gives hope when it seems things are overwhelming – it's empowering to volunteer.'*

So don't reach for the Valium, reach for the mouse. Try do-it.org.uk, join the Carbon Army and help plant a Community Orchard in your town. If you're in need of a shot of grown-up glamour, be a guide at Somerset House for London Fashion Week or hang out at Bryant Park for New York's. Pap the weirdest outfits and post them on *The Sartorialist* (the sartorialist.blogspot.com). If you're over 50 or retired, go to csv-org.uk and use your years of expertise to help others. Bottle-feed orphaned lion cubs in Zambia, track jaguars in Brazil or help restore a medieval castle in the Czech Republic. Just fantasizing about it will make you feel better! For volunteer vacations, visit charityguide.org or read Pam Grout's *The 100 Best Volunteer Vacations*. As singer and activist Joan Baez says, *'Action is the antidote to despair.'*

Susan Sarandon says, 'A lot of what we don't like aesthetically about women who are fighting ageing is fear manifesting. I don't think you should try to look twenty when you are in your sixties. There is something odd about a woman who looks younger than she did twenty years ago.'

'I'VE NO REGRETS. I WOULDN'T HAVE LIVED MY LIFE THE WAY I DID IF I WAS GOING TO WORRY ABOUT WHAT PEOPLE WERE GOING TO SAY.'

INGRID BERGMAN

SEX IS BETTER *(If You Want It!)*

When you're a kidult your worth is very much bound up with your sexuality and the ability to perform theatrically in bed, bus shelter or biscuit factory at the drop of a hat. YouTube, Facebook and Bebo abound with snaps of lithe, smooth bodies contorting for the camera, a carrier bag of Rampant Rabbits close at hand. Headboards bounce against motel walls, high-pitched squeals deafen colonies of bats and a night isn't considered sexy without several sweaty couplings. Us grown-up girls have a little secret – we know it's not the quantity but the quality of our sexual encounters that matters. Orgasmic yodelling probably means one is not concentrating on the job in hand (so to speak) – men take heed! And we are now confident in our own ability to know what really works.

But what if you don't want to do it any more? Well, you may agree with Bette Davis, who described sex as 'God's great joke on human beings' – unlike Mae West who insisted, *'An orgasm a day keeps the doctor away.'* For me, a life without sex might be safer, but also a teensy bit dull. I've always believed love is the answer, but like Woody Allen, I reckon sex raises some damn good questions!

Don't **BE SCARED**

As Cate Blanchett says, *'If you're going to fail, fail gloriously,'* and take heed of Katharine Hepburn's words, 'If you obey all the rules, you miss all the fun.' Just don't be scared! The rules you break don't have to be big at first, you can enjoy little ones – Jerry Hall plans to 'keep wearing bikinis until I'm 80!'

Woman's greatest enemy is insecurity and how we deal with it rather determines how successfully we run our lives as grown-up girls. For instance, if you've been with your partner forever and it's still working out – fabulous! If not, and you feel trapped in a lacklustre relationship, then you can let go – it's a slow death living with someone just because they help pay the bills. Just consider some of the neurotic lives of football WAGs. First and foremost, your key relationship should be with yourself and others second, but that doesn't make you monstrously selfish, probably nicer to be around and thus more pleasurable to be with for others. As Carrie Bradshaw in *Sex and the City* once wrote: 'There are those that open you up to something new and exotic, those that are old and familiar, those that bring up lots of questions, those that bring you somewhere unexpected, those that bring you far from where you started, and those that bring you back. But the most exciting, challenging and significant relationship of all is the one you have with yourself. And if you can find someone to love the you, you love – well, that's just fabulous.'

TAKE A *Deep Breath*

OK, you might think I've flipped, but meditating really does help. It's good for stress and blood pressure – some say it even lowers your biological age, so set aside at least ten minutes every day to just breathe. Here's what to do to improve your karma:

★ Choose somewhere quiet. You don't have to sit cross-legged on the floor – you can be upright in a chair, just as long as you're relaxed.

★ Place your left hand palm-up in your right hand and breathe normally.

★ Count each breath in and out as one, until you get to ten. If you lose track, don't stress – start at one again.

★ Continue until all you are focusing on is your breathing. Ignore the stressed-out machinations of your mind, enjoy the peace and quiet.

Kim Novak says: '*Storms come down, houses are wiped out, people drown, but every last little palm is there after the storm. Man is always saying, "I will overwhelm." Why can't he bend like the little palms and rise again? Isn't that better than being washed away?*'

IT'S A LAUGH, *Innit?*

At the age of 83, Katharine Hepburn – who stood
on her head every day after her daily dive in the lake
– said: 'I think everything's quite funny. Laughing
is fun and I laugh at practically anything.' With
this, I heartily concur. It sounds banal but a good
belly laugh really does make you feel better. It also
strengthens your immune system, exercises the
diaphragm and improves circulation. Laughter helps
with stress and makes you new friends – it's the
most enjoyable form of exercise, full stop. So, try a
bit of laughter therapy. It's easy, if a bit weird when
you start, but trust me:
I do it and it works.

With a partner, offspring or like-minded friend,
just start laughing. Of course the laughter is fake at
first but you'll find this is what makes it funny. Very
quickly you'll be laughing in reality, the tears will
flow and you'll find it hard to stop. I can't tell you
how much better you will feel afterwards.

HOW TO LIVE LIFE
Like a Glamorous Grown-Up

When **CLAUDETTE COLBERT** was in her seventies a reporter asked her: 'What keeps you looking and feeling so young?' She answered smoothly, 'Not worrying about looking and feeling so young!'

SOPHIA LOREN says, 'There is a fountain of youth; it is your mind, your talents, the creativity you bring to your life and the lives of the people you love. When you learn to tap this source, you will truly have defeated age.'

LAUREN BACALL insisted defiantly: '*I'm not a has been, I am a will be.*'

'It's a great age to be. You can do things that are completely off the wall!' said **ELIZABETH TAYLOR** at 60.

MAYA ANGELOU waxes poetic: 'When I passed 40 I dropped pretence, 'cause men like women who got some sense.'

'I actually look forward to getting older – it is certainly better than the alternative; when looks should become less of an issue, and when who you are is the point,' says **SUSAN SARANDON**.

Of course, as **SOPHIE TUCKER** says: '*The secret of longevity is to keep breathing.*'

'I have been uncompromising, peppery, intractable, monomaniacal, tactless, volatile, and oftentimes disagreeable... I suppose I'm larger than life,' observed **BETTE DAVIS**.

Or try **JERRY HALL**'s approach: *'I will grow old gracefully in public – and disgracefully in private.'*

And finally, live like **JANE BIRKIN**: 'Never stop your passion, just keep going. Be modest. Seek great experiences. Be useful. Stick up for what you believe in. Get angry about what you care about.'

'When you're into the second half of your life you really do have to live in a place of acceptance and celebration that you're still here, and being grateful for everything that you have. You begin to see your blessings really.'
MICHELLE PFEIFFER

'Your twenties are torture, really, because you don't know what you are going to be or whether it's all going to work out, and you are supposedly an adult but you haven't really learnt anything. You're always looking for your own place in the world, but you're insecure – you think you're wonderful one minute and you think you're a disaster the next.' And her sixties? 'It's brilliant, really, the way life organizes itself, because you just slowly get used to what you are, don't you?'
HELEN MIRREN

'One day your life will flash before your eyes. Make sure it's worth watching.' **ANON**

'After all these years, I am still involved in the process of self-discovery. It's better to explore life and make mistakes than to play it safe. Mistakes are part of the dues one pays for a full life.' says Sophia Loren.

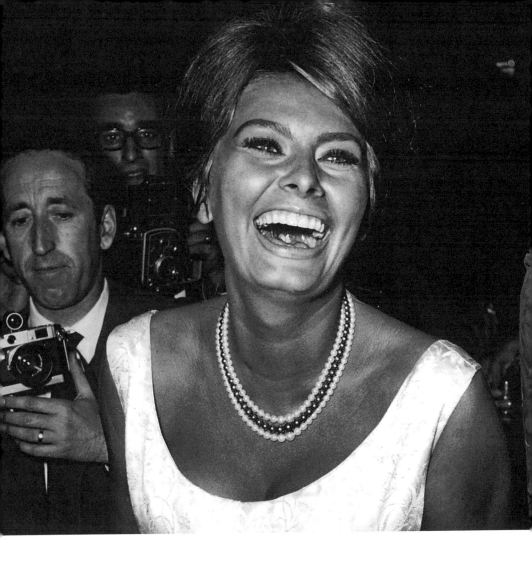

REFERENCES

p.7 Katharine Hepburn in imdb.com/name/nm0000031/bio

p.12 Vivienne Westwood in interview with BBC London Radio, 9 Feb, 2010

p.19 Coco Chanel in *The New Yorker*, Vol 64, 1989 p.75

p.20 Mary Quant in *Colour by Quant*, (New York: McGraw-Hill, 1985) p.122

p.20 Grace Coddington in Amy Hofman Edelman, *The Little Black Dress*, (New York: Simon and Schuster Editions, 1997) p.142

p.23 Marlene Dietrich, *Marlene Dietrich's ABC* (New York: Frederick Ungar Publishing Co., 1961) pp. 48-49

p.24 Carrie Bradshaw in *Sex and the City*, (HBO Season 4, Episode 1, 'The Agony and the Ex'tasy.'

p.25 Coco Chanel in Linda Grant, 'Coco Chanel – la dame aux camelias' in the *Daily Telegraph* 29 July, 2007

p.32 'Fashion: The Main Line' in *Time*, Sept. 27, 1963

p.34 Jackie Onassis in Oleg Cassini, *A Thousand days of Magic: Dressing Jacqueline Kennedy for the White House*, (New York: Rizzoli International, 1995) p.103

p.37 Bill Blass in billblass.com

p.37 Georgia May Jagger in 'Georgia May Jagger: Why Mick's baby girl rocks' in *The Daily Mail*, 21 Aug, 2008

p.41 Mainbocher in brainyquote.com/quotes/authors/m/mainbocher.html

Mainbocher in ibid

Mainbocher in 'Fashion: The Main Line' in *Time*, Sept. 27, 1963

p.47 Marnie Fogg, *Vintage Handbags* (London: Carlton Books, 2009) pp.211-213

p.51 Carrie Bradshaw in *Sex and the City* (HBO Season 3, Episode 17, What Goes Around, Comes Around.'

p.52 Mimi Spencer in Valerie Steele and Laird Borelli, *Bags: A Lexicon of Style* (London: Scriptum Editions, 1999) p.10

p.54 Chloe Sevigny in marieclaire.com/hair-beauty/trends/celebrity-tips/chloe-sevigny-beauty

p.58 Jane Birkin in fashionchronicles.com/handbags/hermes-birkin

p.58 Kelly Brook in *Metro*, 17 March, 2010

p.59 Marie Helvin in 'Me and my wardrobe: Why Marie Helvin is done with her designer clothes' in *The Daily Mail*, 3 Dec, 2009

p.60 Bette Midler in 'Happy Feet!' in *The Calcutta Telegraph*, Feb 16, 2010

p.62 Sarah Jessica Parker in '10 Soleful Questions' in *Time*, 7 Feb, 2003

p.64 Emma Thompson in the *Daily Mirror*, 22 March, 2010

p.65 Helena Christensen in brainyquote.com/quotes/authors/h/helena_christensen.html

Meg Ryan in brainyquote.com/quotes/authors/m/meg_ryan.html

ElleMacpherson in easylivingmagazine.com/RealLife/CelebrityInterview/ElleMacpherson/default.aspx

Rachel Weisz in indexmagazine.com/interviews/rachel_weisz.shtml

p.66 Sophia Loren, *Women & Beauty* (London: Aurum Press, 1984) p.109

p.69 Twiggy in Twiggy: My fashion secrets, *The Daily Mail*, 19th Sept, 2008

p.69 Michel de Montaigne, *The Complete Essays* (London: Penguin Classic, 1993) p.98

p.72 Britt Ekland, *Sensual Beauty and How to Achieve It* (London:

Sidgwick & Jackson, 1983) p.120

p.75 Sophia Loren, *Women & Beauty* (London: Aurum Press, 1984) pp.109-110

p.75 Marlene Dietrich, *Marlene Dietrich's ABC* (New York: Frederick Ungar Publishing Co., 1961) p.67

p.79 Joan Rivers in saidwhat.co.uk/quotes/favourite/joan_rivers

p.80 norway.org.uk/business/news/voss.htm

p.82 Pamela Anderson in Sherryl Connelly, 'Pamela Anderson hits the beach sans sunscreen and claims 'nothing's been shot into this face' *New York Daily News*, 10 Sept, 2009

p.83 Noel Coward, *Play Parade* (New York: Garden City Publishing, 1933) p.39

p.86 Professor Chris Griffiths in sawfnews.com/health/35311.aspx

p.90 Jennifer Aniston in ivillage.co.uk/newspol/celeb/cint/articles/0,,528729_711781,00.html

p.90 Penelope Cruz in Roger Dobson, 'Can too much sleep be bad for your body?; 'For Penelope Cruz, nothing less than 15 hours will do. But too much sleep can make many people miserable and depressed.' *The London Evening Standard*, Feb 12, 2002

p.90 Halle Berry in *People*, March 16, 2008

p.90 Nigella Lawson in 'How Nigella Lawson won the ageing game' in *The Sydney Morning Herald*, Nov 17, 2008

p.90 Teri Hatcher in ibid

p.93 Claudia Schiffer in celebritybeautybuzz.com/index.php/category/claudia-schiffer/

Estee Lauder in esteelauder.co.uk

Iman in Beth Neil, 'Fifty. It's the new phwoarty' in *Daily Mirror*, 23 Jan, 201

Sharon Stone in 'Stone age: sassier and more honest than ever, Sharon Stone is now the face of Dior's new skincare line' in *W*, Feb 1, 2006

Cate Blanchett in marieclaire.com/hair-beauty/trends/celebrity-tips/cate-blanchett-beauty-routine

Coco Chanel in *Coco Chanel: her life, her secrets* (London: Hale, 1972) p.153

(Caption) Iman in rollingout.com/insideentertainment/the-pulse/979-iman-putting-her-best-face-forward-.html

p.94 Kate Winslet in celebritybeautybuzz.com/index.php/category/kate-winslet/

John Galliano in 'Treatment of the Week' in *The Daily Mail*, Mar 8, 2010

p.96 (Caption) Christy Turlington in Joan Juliet Buck, 'Beauty and Soul,' *Vogue*, August, 2009

p.98 Nora Ephron in Janet Maslin, 'Oh, the Indignity: Nora Ephron Confronts Ageing and Other New York Battles' in *The New York Times*, July 27, 2006

p.100 Susan Sarandon in *The Orange County Register*, June 6, 2008

Susan Penhaligon in Anita Singh, 'Fouled Botox creates 'monsters' ' in *New Zealand Herald on Sunday*, Jan 3, 2010

p.101 Susan Sarandon in imdb.com/name/nm0000215/bio

Rosanna Arquette in brainyquote.com

Kate Winslet in http://specialkatewinslet.blogspot.com/

Catherine Deneuve in Lisa Armstrong, 'Catherine, the great survivor' in *The Times*, Aug 1, 2007

Cate Blanchett in andhranews.net/Entertainment/2008/May/13-

Cate-Blanchett-refuses-44598.asp
Halle Berry in 'Halle Berry Interview: Closer to Home' in *Reader's Digest*, April 2007
Jennifer Aniston in 'Face to Face with Jennifer Aniston' *Elle* UK April 2009
Teri Hatcher in *Glamour*, March 2007
p.102 Sharon Osbourne in 'Nipped, tucked and talking' *People*, Sep 2, 2003
Janice Dickinson in allgreatquotes.com/plastic_surgery_quotes.shtml
Linda Evans in icelebz.com/quotes/linda_evans/
Sadie Frost in 'This Body is 100 per cent real' in *Grazia*, 11 Jan, 2010
Jerry Hall in Alison Roberts, 'I'm sick of the toyboys' *The London Evening Standard*, 14 May, 2007
p.106 Yves Saint Laurent in goodreads.com/quotes/show/28802
Bette Davis in bettedavis.com/about/quotes.htm
Sandra Bullock in tv.com/sandra-bullock/person/43646/trivia.html
Calvin Klein in brainyquote.com/quotes/authors/c/calvin_klein_3.html
Lauren Hutton in interview, CNN Live Today, Oct 3, 2003
Helena Rubenstein in atozquotes.com/authors/author_12404
Daniel Kolaric in interview with author, 2 Dec 2009
p.111 Sharon Stone in celebritywonder.com/html/sharonstone_trivia1.html
p.114 Daniel Kolaric in interview with author, 2 Dec, 2009
p.117 Sarah Jessica Parker in celebritybeautybuzz.com/index.php/2010/01/sarah-jessica-parkers-5-favorite-beauty-products/
p.121 Mala Rubenstein, *The Mala Rubenstein Book of Beauty* (London: Angus & Robertson, 1974) pp.8-9
p.126 Jerry Seinfeld in http://zikkir.com/content/72507
Lauren Hutton in laurenhutton.com/about-good-stuff.html
p.129 Cate Blanchett in http://thebeautybunny.com/cate-blanchett-what-makeup-does-she-use/
p.130 Lana Turner in quotesdaddy.com/author/Lana+Turner
p.131 Carole Lombard in 'Carole Lombard Tells: 'How I Live By a Man's Code' in *Photoplay* no. 51, June 1937
p.135 Hubert de Givenchy in *Vogue*, July 1985
p.136 Edward Darley in interview with author, Feb 12, 2010
p.137 Ibid
p.142 Diane von Furstenberg, *Diane von Furstenberg's Book of Beauty: How to become a more attractive, confident and sensual woman* (New York: Simon and Schuster, 1976) pp.114-5
p. 149 Marie Helvin in *Now*, Aug 31, 2006
p.152 Britt Ekland, *Sensual Beauty and How to Achieve It* (London: Sidwick & Jackson, 1983) p.41
p.153 Jerry Hall in Beth Neil, 'Fifty. It's the new phwoarty' in *Daily Mirror*, 23 Jan, 2010
p.157 Helen Mirren in http://allgreatquotes.com/helen_mirren_quotes.shtml
p.159 Helen Mirren in *The Daily Record*, Jan 13, 2010
Jason Fraser in *The Independent*, 28 July, 2008
p.160 Kathleen Turner, *Send Yourself Roses: My Life, Loves and Leading Roles* (London: Headline Publishing, 2008) p. 178
p.163 (Caption) Michelle Obama in *The Huffington Post*, March 6, 2009
p.165 Tilda Swinton in *The Daily Mail*, 14 Feb 2008
(Caption) Tilda Swinton in dailymail.co.uk/femail/article-515159/How-Tilda-Swinton-stole-boyfriend-m-eacute-nage-agrave-trois.html
p.167 Tallulah Bankhead in *The New York Times*, Dec 13, 1968
- in Alex Madsen, *The Sewing Circle* (New York: Birch Lane Press, 1995) p.118
- in *Financial Times*, July 2, 1997
- in workinghumor.com/quotes/tallulah_bankhead.shtml
in brainyquote.com/quotes/authors/t/tallulah_bankhead.html
in imdb.com/name/nm0000845/bio
in goodreads.com/quotes/show/207382
in goodreads.com/author/quotes/373655.Tallulah_Bankhead
in ibid
p.168 (Caption) Jessica Vartoughian in 'Jessica Vartoughian – as hard as nails' *The London Evening Standard*, Jan 27, 2010
p.169 Barbra Streisand in contactmusic.com/new/xmlfeed.nsf/story/streisand.-.fingernails-brought-me-fame.
p.170 Joan Crawford in *Film Pictorial*, 30 Sept, 1933
p.172 Vivienne Westwood in *The Daily Mail*, June 9, 2006 (all quotes)
p.173 Frank Sinatra in Kitty Kelley, *His Way: the unauthorized biography of Frank Sinatra* (New York: Bantam Press, 1986) p.165
Shelley Winters in brainyquote.com/quotes/keywords/overweight.html
In *Marie Claire*, Jan 2007
In filmbug.com/db/31297/quotes
p.174 Bill Blanko, 'Lumley charms the drooling classes' in *The Guardian*, 7 May, 2009
Joanna Lumley in Laura Barton, 'I don't make a very good goddess' *The Guardian*, 31 Aug, 2009
- ibid
- ibid
- ibid
p.178 Jackie Onassis in *The New York Times*, 20 May, 1994
- Roswell Gilpatric in Shelley Branch and Sue Calloway, *What would Jackie Do?* (New York: Gotham Books, 2007) p.168
p.179 Marlene Dietrich, *Marlene Dietrich's ABC* (New York: Frederick Ungar Publishing Co., 1961) p.33
p.187 Freya Stark, *The Journey's Echo* (New York: Harcourt, Brace & World) 1964 p. 199
p.193 Reid Buckley in *National Review*, 16 April, 1990
p.194 Colette in James M. Markham, 'St Tropez Journal: Tourist Throngs Overshadow a Place in the Sun' *The New York Times*, 19 Aug, 1987
p.196 Marlene Dietrich, *Marlene Dietrich's ABC* (New York: Frederick Ungar Publishing Co., 1961) p.159
- Orson Welles in worldbackpackers.net/travel-quotes/
p.197 Britt Ekland, *Sensual Beauty and How to Achieve It* (London: Sidwick & Jackson, 1983) p.132
- Margaret Mead in Mary C. Fjeldstad, *The Thoughtful Reader* (Fort Worth: Harcourt Brace College Publishers, 1998) p.48
- Scott Donaldson, *The Cambridge Companion to Hemingway* (Cambridge: Cambridge University press, 1996) p.216

251

p.203 Michelle Obama in 'Michelle Obama shares dating secrets: 'Cute only lasts for so long.' *New York Daily News*, Oct 28 2009
- Drew Barrymore, Interview on CBS Early Show, Feb 2 2009
(caption) Demi Moore in Laura Brown, 'Demi Moore's Dream Life: The Interview. *Harper's Bazaar*, April 2010
p.204 Demi Moore in Kevin West, 'Demi Goddess' in *W* Dec 2009
- Courtney Cox in eatsleepcelebrity.com/2010/03/courteney-cox-arquette-is-a-real-cougar/
p.205 Sophia Loren, *Women & Beauty* (London: Aurum Press, 1984) p.166
p.206 Iman in intermix.org.uk/relationships/couples_david_and_iman.asp
p.207 Phoebe in *Friends*, Season 2, Episode 14, 'The One with the Prom Video.'
- Courtney Cox in showbizspy.com/article/190849/courteney-cox-gives-dating-tips.html
- Joseph Weintraub (ed) *The Wit and Wisdom of Mae West* (New York: Avon, 1970) p.87
p.213 Katherine Heigl in http://entertainment.stv.tv/film/130979-katherine-heigls-sexy-date-outfits/
p.214 Clark Gable in imdb.com/name/nm0000022/bio
p.218 Jennifer Lopez in brainyquote.com/quotes/authors/j/jennifer_lopez.html
- Mistinguett in Tomima Edmark, *Kissing: Everything You Ever Wanted to Know* (London: Prentice-Hall, 1991) p.29
- Ingrid Bergman in ingridbergman.com/about/quotes.htm
- Katherine Heigl in squidoo.com/Katherine_Heigl
- Heidi Klum in http://us.hadnews.com/heidi-klum-seal-is-a-supersexy-hot-kisser.htm
- Joseph Weintraub (ed) *The Wit and Wisdom of Mae West* (New York: Avon, 1970) p.79
- Kim Cattrall as Samantha in *Sex and the City*, (HBO Season 1, Episode 6, 'Secret Sex.'
p.221 Marlene Dietrich, *Marlene Dietrich's ABC* (New York: Frederick Ungar Publishing Co., 1961) p.49
- (caption) Marlene Dietrich in Jeannie Williams 'Gossip, Gossip and More Gossip' *New York* magazine, Aug 1 1994
p.225 Nigella Lawson in *Esquire*, Nov 2007
p.227 Elle Macpherson in easylivingmagazine.com/RealLife/CelebrityInterview/ElleMacpherson/default.aspx
- Bette Davis in http://womenshistory.about.com/od/quotes/a/bette_davis.htm
p.230 (Caption) *The New York Times*, May 18 1966
p.235 Tilda Swinton in Gaby Wood, 'Tilda Opens Up' *The Guardian*, Oct 9, 2005
p.236 Gloria Swanson in Gina Lollobrigida, *The Wonder of Innocence* (Harry H. Abrams, 1994) p.49
- Eva Gabor in Allison Vale & Alison Rattle, *More Wrinklies' Wit and Wisdom* (London: Sevenoaks, 2006) p.114
p.237 Meg Ryan in meg-ryan.net/library-lifeofmegryan.php
p.238 Britt Ekland in *Sensual Beauty and How to Achieve It* (London: Sidwick & Jackson, 1983) p.7
p.241 Susan Sarandon in http://women.webmd.com/features/susan-sarandon
- (Caption) Susan Sarandon in Chrissy Illey 'Susan Sarandon: sexy, single and 63' *The Observer*, 17 Jan, 2010
p.243 Bette Davis and Mickey Herskowitz, *This n' That* (New York: Putnam, 1987) p.67
- Mae West in George Eells, Stanley Musgrove, *Mae West: a biography* (New York: William Morrow & Co. 1982) p.12
p.244 Cate Blanchett in imdb.com/name/nm0000949/bio
- Jerry Hall in Allison Vale & Alison Rattle, *More Wrinklies' Wit and Wisdom* (London: Sevenoaks, 2006) p.53
- Carrie Bradshaw in *Sex and the City*, (HBO Season 6, Episode 20, 'An American Girl in Paris: Part Deux.'
p.245 Kim Novak in quotelucy.com/keywords/storm-quotes.html
p.247 Claudette Colbert in Earl Blackwell, *Earl Blackwell's Celebrity Register* (Michigan: Gale Group, 1990) p.103
- Sophia Loren in Allison Vale & Alison Rattle, *More Wrinklies' Wit and Wisdom* (London: Sevenoaks, 2006) p.84
- Lauren Bacall in brainyquote.com/quotes/quotes/l/laurenbaca104647.html
- Elizabeth Taylor in Allison Vale & Alison Rattle, *More Wrinklies' Wit and Wisdom* (London: Sevenoaks, 2006) p.70
- May Angelou in Ibid, p.50
- Susan Sarandon in http://celebrifi.com/gossip/Kate-Hudson-MaryKate-Olsen-Susan-Sarandon-SemiNude-Photos-Hollywood-Pinups-Book-181757.html
- Sophie Tucker in Allison Vale & Alison Rattle, *More Wrinklies' Wit and Wisdom* (London: Sevenoaks, 2006) p.82
- Bette Davis, *The Lonely Life: an autobiography* (New York: Putnam, 1962) p.245
p.248 Jerry Hall in Allison Vale & Alison Rattle, *More Wrinklies' Wit and Wisdom* (London: Sevenoaks, 2006) p.53
- Jane Birkin in squidoo.com/whatdoiwear
- Michelle Pfeiffer in *The Telegraph*, 20 April, 2009
- Helen Mirren in Simon Hattenstone, 'Nothing Like a Dame' *The Guardian*, 2 Sept, 2006
(Caption) Sophia Loren in sophialoren.org/more.html

Every effort has been made to contact the copyright holders of text included in this book in order to obtain permission to reproduce extracts and adaptations of copyright material. For further information, please contact Quadrille Publishing Ltd.

INDEX

Acknowledgements

To the glamorous grown-ups Anne Furniss, Marnie Fogg, Maggie Norden, Khalid Siddiqui, literary agent Sheila Ableman, Clive Ball, Edward Darley and all at Sassoon Academy, Daniel Kolaric, Katey Mackenzie, Claire Peters, Emma Sanders, Tina Haukjaer Andersen for her insider knowledge of vintage Los Angeles, Laurie and Chris for their help in a Mac crisis, Ann and Alan Carter for their enthusiasm and support – and the ever-wonderful Lionel Marsden.

Editorial director Anne Furniss
Creative director Helen Lewis
Editor Katey Mackenzie
Designer Claire Peters
Picture assistant Samantha Rolfe
Production director Vincent Smith
Production controller Ruth Deary

First published in 2010 by
Quadrille Publishing Ltd
Alhambra House
27–31 Charing Cross Road
London WC2H 0LS
www.quadrille.co.uk

British Library Cataloguing-in-Publication Data
A catalogue record for this book is available from the British Library.

ISBN: 978 1 84400 887 2

Printed in China

PICTURE CREDITS 4 Michael Ochs Archives/Getty Images; 17 Alex Oliveira/Rex Features; 18 Eamonn McCormack/WireImage/Getty Images; 28 ©Bettmann/CORBIS; 35 Ron Galella/WireImage/Getty Images; 36 Ron Galella/WireImage/Getty Images; 48 Reg Burkett/Hulton Collection/Getty Images; 55 Ben King/Rex Features; 56 Eric Ryan/Getty Images; 63 Everett Collection/Rex Feature; 73 Arnaldo Magnani/Getty Images; 74 Andrew H. Walker/Getty Images; 85 ©Nicolas Tikhomiroff/Magnum Photos; 91 Picture Perfect/Rex Features; 92 Sipa Press/Rex Features; p97 ©Martine Franck/Magnum Photos; 109 BDG/Rex Features; 118 ©Underwood & Underwood/CORBIS; 127 Gabriel Bouys/AFP/Getty Images; 128 Bruce Glikas/FilmMagic/Getty Images; 138 Warner Bros/Everett Collection/Rex Features; 145 R. Hepler/Everett/Rex Features; 146 Everett Collection/Rex Feature; 163 ©Joyce N. Boghosian/White House/Handout/CNP/Corbis; 164 Jeff Vespa/VF/WireImage/Getty Images; 168 Everett Collection/Rex Feature; 183 Hulton Archive/Getty Images; 184 ©Eve Arnold/Magnum Photos; 191 SNAP/Rex Features; 201 ©Bettmann/CORBIS; 202 John Parra/WireImage/Getty Images; 219 ©Mario Anzuoni/Reuters/Corbis; 220 Everett Collection/Rex Features; 231 Hulton Archive/Getty Images; 239 UMDADC/Rex Features; 240 ©Mike Giro./Retna Ltd./Corbis; 249 LYNX/Rex Features.